ORDINARY MIRACLES

*Learning from Breast
Cancer Survivors*

S. David Nathanson, M.D.
with David Stringer

The Praeger Series on Contemporary Health and Living
Julie Silver, Series Editor

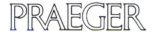

Westport, Connecticut
London

Library of Congress Cataloging-in-Publication Data

Nathanson, S. David.
Ordinary miracles : learning from breast cancer survivors / S. David Nathanson
with David Stringer.
     p.   cm.—(The Praeger series on contemporary health and living, ISSN 1932–8079)
     Includes bibliographical references and index.
     ISBN-13: 978–0–275–99469–3 (alk. paper)
     ISBN-10: 0–275–99469–4 (alk. paper)
     1. Breast—Cancer—Patients—Portraits.   2. Breast—Cancer—Patients—Anecdotes.
     I. Title.   II. Series.
     [DNLM: 1. Breast Neoplasms—psychology—Personal Narratives.   2. Survivors—
     psychology—Personal Narratives.   WP 870 N275o 2007]
  RC280.B8O7337   2007
  362.196′9944900922—dc22   2007008451

British Library Cataloguing in Publication Data is available.

Library of Congress Catalog Card Number: 2007008451
ISBN-13: 978–0–275–99469–3
ISBN-10: 0–275–99469–4
ISSN: 1932–8079

First published in 2007

Praeger Publishers, 88 Post Road West, Westport, CT 06881
An imprint of Greenwood Publishing Group, Inc.
www.praeger.com

Printed in the United States of America

The paper used in this book complies with the
Permanent Paper Standard issued by the National
Information Standards Organization (Z39.48–1984).

10 9 8 7 6 5 4 3 2 1

This book is for general information only. No book can ever substitute for the judgment of a
medical professional. If you have worries or concerns, contact your doctor.

Some of the names and details of individual discussed in this book have been changed to protect
the patients' identities. Some of the stories may be composites of patient interactions created for
illustrative purposes.

CONTENTS

SERIES FOREWORD

Over the past hundred years, there have been incredible medical break-throughs that have prevented or cured illness in billions of people and helped many more improve their health while living with chronic conditions. A few of the most important twentieth-century discoveries include antibiotics, organ transplants, and vaccines. The twenty-first century has already heralded important new treatments including such things as a vaccine to prevent human papillomavirus from infecting and potentially leading to cervical cancer in women. Polio is on the verge of being eradicated worldwide, making it only the second infectious disease behind smallpox to ever be erased as a human health threat.

In this series, experts from many disciplines share with readers important and updated medical knowledge. All aspects of health are considered including subjects that are disease-specific and preventive medical care. Disseminating this information will help individuals to improve their health as well as researchers to determine where there are gaps in our current knowledge and policy-makers to assess the most pressing needs in health care.

Series Editor Julie Silver, M.D.
Assistant Professor
Harvard Medical School
Department of Physical Medicine and Rehabiliation

ACKNOWLEDGMENTS

My patients inspired this book. Many of them are found within its pages. Many more created lasting memories and images in my mind. I am grateful that they allowed me to manage their medical problems and to share their emotions, fears, and experiences.

I've been lucky enough to work with great doctors, scientists, and teachers. I've spent most of my career as a breast surgeon at Henry Ford Health System in Detroit, Michigan. My many colleagues in Radiology, Pathology, Medical Oncology, Radiation Oncology, and General Surgical, too numerous to name individually, have provided the depth and meaning to my career that allowed me to compile the book.

Patients would be lost without nurses. Wanda Szymanski, R.N., is singled out by many patients for her style; she has been a pillar of strength to me too. Milica Kay, R.N., Debbie McEvoy, R.N., and Joan Evans, R.N., all provided immeasurable help to patients and to the physicians they work with. My patients and I have benefited from many other nurses; women who've provided compassionate care to my patients include Sue, Suzie, Paula, Karen, Florence, Michelle, Lisa, Lorraine, Debbie, and Latoya.

Most women cope well with the behavioral and social aspects of their breast cancers but we have all benefited from the "altruistic angels," the social workers and nurse practitioners who help patients navigate the psychological, social, and other aspects of their lives after receiving a diagnosis of breast cancer. Occasionally patients need more than they can get from family, physicians, nurses, and friends; Wendy Goldberg, whose awe-inspiring personal experiences with her own disease in Chapter 10 give us an intimate view of a magnificent woman, is the "go to" person for those who need help in managing the stress of their disease.

Sally Cole-Saul, whose stories are visible in many of the chapters, inspired me from the beginning. Her unswerving optimism provided me the energy I needed to start this project. Linda D'Antonio, whose personal saga is in

Chapter 12, has provided the tenacity, energy, and inspiration that I needed to continue with the project.

I met David Stringer, a retired high-school English teacher from Saline, Michigan, over lunch in August 2005. We had an animated discussion about what I needed and we quickly came to a "meeting of the minds." He very rapidly put all the patients' stories into a readable format. I gave him the outline for the chapters and he expertly edited, collated, and filled those chapters. I provided bridging ideas and he provided the appropriate grammatical and editorial skills that an English teacher knows so well.

Without the facilities provided by the Henry Ford Health System we would not have had the opportunity to see the thousands of patients over the almost 20 years that we've run a Multidisciplinary Breast Cancer Program. The administration, coordination, funding, and quality of our program would not have been possible without the strong support we received from the Chief Executive Officer, the Chief Medical Officer, the Director of the Cancer Center, Department Chairs, Division Chiefs, clerks, data managers, secretaries, research nurses, Cancer Coordinators, and our generous hardworking hospital staff.

My mentors and teachers from medical school, surgical residencies, and fellowship training were great role models. From them I learned to listen to the patient. I believe that the most important aspect of patient care is to be a healer. Healers don't preach or intimidate. Healers don't rush off somewhere else until they've helped their patient through the often stressful quagmire initiated by the discovery of an unpleasant diagnosis; they provide a safe haven to people who are ill and need calm strength. I'm grateful that my teachers taught me this important message. Gratefulness is an important attitude, an approach to life that is indispensable to anyone who aspires to wholeness. This I learned from Brother David Steindl-Rast, a Benedictine monk, whose piety, wisdom, and sacredness transformed my own life and whose organization (www.gratefulness.org) is a resource for us all.

My wife and children have stood by me and I can never thank them enough for their love and devotion.

I was fortunate enough to attend Dr. Julie Silver's writing course at Harvard Medical School. There I met Debbie Carvalko from Praeger and she and her staff have helped me through the publication process, gently steering me in the right direction.

Of course there is an invisible guiding light, an energy that helps us through all of our tasks in this world and without which I would be lost.

Introduction: How and Why We Wrote This Book

Clear-eyed hope gives us courage to confront our circumstances and the capacity to surmount them.

—Jerome Groopman, *The Anatomy of Hope: How People Prevail in the Face of Illness* (2004)

You can either be bitter or better.

—advice given by her family doctor to a patient facing a debilitating chronic disease

Why write about the personal experiences and feelings of breast cancer patients? I had not intended to write a book about feelings and emotions. After all, I am a surgeon and scientist, not a psychiatrist.

I often tell new breast cancer patients stories about other patients' experiences without revealing names. Each person has her own way of dealing with the diagnosis and management of her breast cancer, but everyone likes to hear stories of other people whose experiences may have been similar to their own. One of my patients was an energetic, optimistic, educated, inquisitive, and highly motivated woman with a newly diagnosed breast cancer. Sally Cole-Saul had her surgery and, just like all my other patients, returned to see me in the office. I continued to see her in follow-up in the usual fashion. Whenever we met in the clinic we would take a few minutes to deal with her medical problems, and many minutes to talk about her work, hobbies, travels, friends, family, and other activities. She was curious about my life and asked questions about my interests and family. I had been taught to evade such questions from patients, but Sally's strength and perseverance would not allow me to hide my personality during our encounters over many years. I began to share some of my personal life with her and, when I discovered this didn't adversely affect our doctor–patient relationship, I felt comfortable in calling her both friend and patient.

One day she asked me when I would be writing a book.

"A book about what?"

"Breast cancer, of course!"

"There are already many types of books on breast cancer. Do you think it is important to write another one?"

"I know that I needed to learn how other women with breast cancer were coping with the diagnosis. You often tell me how patients confide some of their feelings to you. Why don't you write about that? Why don't we ask your patients to share their stories?"

I thanked her and told her I'd think about it. She had planted a seed in my brain that kept growing when I saw other patients. Sally thought that a book written by patients and touching on their relationship with doctors, nurses, family, and friends would be unique, and she enthusiastically offered to help put it together. The result is this book.

Could I ask my patients to share their stories with a wide array of people? Couldn't I just summarize their stories for them, sparing them all the difficulties of confronting and disclosing intimate information? I quickly realized that patients had to tell their own stories. Good storytelling is an art that has evolved over millennia, but not even the best writers can accurately capture the passions of the individual who lived through such a profoundly personal event as breast cancer. Only the patient who has experienced breast cancer treatment knows which deep, meaningful memories are important to her.

Another reason why this book needs to be written by the patients is that 99 percent of breast cancer patients are women, and men cannot interpret, evaluate, or even truly understand the emotions and feelings of women who are treated for breast cancer. My voice in the book needs to constantly admit this truth while commenting on the writings of the patients in each chapter. Knowing that I can at best be a witness to their experience, I have attempted to inform each chapter with this sincere humility.

My experiences in the Multidisciplinary Breast Cancer Clinic have brought me in contact with thousands of patients. Indeed, physicians, nurses, and other health care professionals are daily exposed to rich stories from their patients. People who are ill feel vulnerable and, when they find a medical professional they can trust, often confide deep and intimate stories. I sometimes half jokingly tell medical students, residents in training, and the nurses that work with me that I don't need to read novels because the stories I hear from patients are filled with the same kind of drama, conflict, mystery, and comedy that are found in any well-written fiction. Their stories were unique, rich in feelings, emotions, and experiences, and I was entertained as well as educated. Many of them were sad, but most were filled with humor and love, and occasionally they made me laugh out loud. Sometimes I felt overwhelming sadness when I realized that someone I thought I knew had such painful thoughts without telling me in the clinic.

The process of "opening up" is usually beneficial to patients. Most of them begin without much knowledge of the disease, and they are enormously fearful when they first hear the word "cancer" applied to them. One of our objectives is to help overcome the fear that magnifies feelings of impending pain, suffering, death, loss of control of their lives, and of the unknown. They may feel better simply because they experience compassionate care, which may begin with their finding someone who will listen to their fears and reassure them about the treatment that lies ahead. It takes knowledge as well as courage to overcome fear, and most patients are relieved when they learn that their treatment options will not necessarily cause extreme pain and suffering. The statistics of recovery and cure are very promising and provide a source of optimism that helps overcome fear. Hope inspires courage.

Many breast cancer patients express hope when they realize that there is a strong statistical chance that they will not have to confront this illness again. Hope, as we learned from the eighteenth-century English poet Alexander Pope, "springs eternal from the human breast." I've also seen that patients with no chance of cure live their last remaining months with hope. These patients all went through an initial phase of fear, an understandable feeling that often results in severe anxiety and depression. But the feeling of hope is so strong that most patients overcome the fear. Hope firms up the resilience that enables a patient to go through arduous treatment. Hope initiates the fortitude that we often recognize in patients experiencing multiple treatments.

Using Sally's and my combined experience of physician and patient, we developed a tentative outline. We designed a format for the book that was based on the common time sequences of breast cancer treatment that each patient experiences. I developed a list of 800 breast cancer patients whom I had operated upon over the past 10 years, and I mailed a letter to each of them, asking for their stories. I thought most would respond because patients were so often willing to confide in me in the clinic. I believed it would be cathartic for patients to write down their feelings. The process of identifying and clarifying thoughts and feelings can be transforming for both the writer and reader. As with psychotherapy, describing experiences and feelings affords the individual an opportunity to master strong emotions and increase self-understanding. Besides, I was sure that the patients would want to help others going through the same unpleasant experiences they themselves had survived.

The responses came in slowly, and only from a small fraction of the recipients. Whenever I asked patients directly to send me their responses they either told me that they were reluctant (because they were concerned about confidentiality) or they promised to get to it "soon." In the meantime, the responses from those who thought the project worthwhile ranged from short paragraphs that didn't reveal feelings to detailed essays from highly motivated people who were courageous enough to write everything they could remember.

I felt discouraged by the reticence of my patients to help complete the book, but I was determined to pursue it in a form that would incorporate all the responses. I know that some patients didn't want to relive the pain of their own experiences, and some felt their experiences should remain private. I also realized that the amount of work required was far beyond the capabilities of my dear patients who had volunteered to help put the project together. I turned to professional help, and the work you'll read in this book is the result of a dedicated professional writer, David Stringer, who used his experience and writing skills to work with me to make each of the stories and comments into a cohesive and readable book that emphasizes the most helpful themes and patterns of feelings.

Our effort started with a plan, and it has evolved into a finished product that is a little different from the one I imagined. We generally follow the time sequence beginning with detection and diagnosis and progressing through surgery, radiation, and chemotherapy, with each patient's story divided among these chapters. We also include individual "case studies" that work as unified chapters. Thematic chapters dealing with support systems, spiritual connections, and direct advice from breast cancer survivors to those newly diagnosed with the disease round out the structure of the book.

We decided on *Ordinary Miracles* as the title of the book once we began to work with the stories that the women told. The accounts of survival seem "miraculous" because of the sense of dread associated with the word "cancer," but they are also "ordinary" because the people who survive breast cancer and go on to lead meaningful and happy lives are not superhuman exceptions to the rule. Their strength and courage reside within us all, and in that sense they are ordinary.

Breast cancer is indeed a dreaded disease, sometimes deadly, and many fear that the diagnosis of breast cancer means certain death preceded by suffering inflicted by the treatment as well as the disease. Survival and reemergence into a meaningful life—often more meaningful than before the diagnosis—seems like a miracle. Many cancer patients hopefully cite the story of Lance Armstrong's survival of testicular cancer that had metastasized to his brain, but they also see his story as an indication of his superhuman performance in surviving cancer and winning the Tour de France bicycle race seven times.

For most, however, survival after breast cancer treatment is an *ordinary* miracle. It has been made ordinary through enormous progress in medical research involving diagnosis, surgery, radiation, and chemotherapy, as well as equal progress in understanding how the medical team is not just treating the disease but rather treating the patient as a whole person. In fact, a key performer in this medical team is the patient herself, usually working with family and friends. The success stories of these patients do not depend on superhuman athleticism and luck, but on the very human and universally shared qualities of courage, fortitude, trust, persistence, faith, and hope.

Patients with breast cancer almost always need a surgical operation. They sometimes need chemotherapy, radiation, hormone manipulation, and some other targeted therapy with an evolving collection of "smart" drugs that promise an even higher cure rate than that currently possible. The treatment of this formerly devastating disease has changed drastically over the past 100 years. From radical surgery introduced at the beginning of the twentieth century, with unbelievably agonizing cosmetic and functional effects, we now have operations that are just as effective and cosmetically acceptable. Reconstruction of the breast, when indicated, produces a visually good likeness of the normal breast in most instances. Radiation therapy has evolved from a crude, inexact science to a highly effective technique with minimal side effects. Chemotherapy has advanced from drugs that were highly toxic and always dreaded, to an era of even more effective drugs but with minimal discomfort and sickness because of support therapy that has almost totally eradicated intolerable side effects. Hormone manipulation therapy has become widespread and is tolerated extremely well by most people. The result of these changes, coupled with an earlier diagnosis resulting from screening mammograms, has dramatically increased the cure rate for breast cancer throughout the world. A patient with an early stage breast cancer in 2005 can expect to be alive without a recurrence in 10 years with about 90 percent probability. Hope does "spring eternal from the human breast"—and well it should.

The stories in this book emphasize the ordinary humanity of the women and men who suffer from breast cancer. Health care professionals are usually dedicated and caring, and the results of the treatments they provide may seem miraculous. The strength of cancer survivors is an ordinary human strength, though we may not all know we have it until we are challenged to use it.

These stories are not from patients who are likely to die soon but are rather from and about those patients who have survived initial surgery and other treatments. They do show a range of emotions and feelings, and all are true. We elected to leave the original grammar and storytelling techniques of each patient unchanged, except where changes were necessary for clarification. The names of the individuals who allowed us to publish their thoughts, experiences, and emotions have been rendered in three different formats: full names in those patients who wished to be known fully; in order to protect their privacy, most patients were comfortable with first names or, in those who wanted to remain even more anonymous, we have given them fictitious names.

In the mythological story Pandora receives a box from Zeus. The box contained all human blessings and all human curses. Although she was forbidden to open the box, she was unable to restrain herself and opened it. In an instant all the curses were released into the world, and all the blessings escaped and were lost—except one: hope. Without hope none of us can endure. Hope is an important component of healing. This book brings stories of hope through the personal emotions, experiences, and feelings of real people with breast cancer. We are privileged to witness these stories and to learn from them.

1

Case Study—Pamela Brady: "A Bump in the Road of Life"

The story of Pamela Brady's recovery from breast cancer is in many ways typical of the stories in this book. It's an account of an "ordinary miracle"—a triumph over a dreaded disease by a woman whose vibrant humanity resonates with the best in all of us.

In this first "case study" in the book, Pamela tells her breast cancer story straight through following the format of the questionnaire we designed. Only the names have been changed. She was 55 years old when she discovered her cancer.

Cancer Anniversary—January 19, 2001: How My Breast Cancer Was Discovered

I'd had my yearly physical in September 2000. At that time, my internist did the breast examination and found nothing. I usually got my yearly mammogram very soon afterward since it has to be ordered by a referring physician. I was unusually busy and when I got around to making the appointment, and the waiting time was 2 months. I got the mammogram in November and was called about 5 days later to come in for a recheck, the staff person saying that the radiologist saw something but in almost all cases it didn't mean anything was wrong, so don't worry. I'd been getting yearly mammograms for almost 20 years and nothing like this had ever happened to me before. I thought to myself, "I won't worry. I'll get it rechecked right now." I told the receptionist, "Fine, I could come down this afternoon." Hah! The soonest she could get me in was 25 days. Did she know that there are 24 hours in each of those days and 60 minutes in each of those hours? I think I felt every one of them. I got an incredible amount of housework done in those 25 days, doing anything and everything to keep busy and not think about that report.

The calendar dragged and hardly a moment went by without a gnawing awareness of this uncertainty in the recesses of my mind. I was on hold, biding time until the recheck mammogram. Along with the recheck came a biopsy and visit with a surgeon who took over control of my case from the radiologist. Since I was always very similar medically and systematically to my older sister who had cysts, I was certain the same would be said of me. It wasn't. The surgeon hurried the test results since we were leaving for a 31-day visit to New Zealand, meeting my sister and her husband there in the middle of their 3-month celebration of her retirement after 40 years of teaching. Asking us to drop by his office on the way to the airport, the surgeon must have been really optimistic about the amount of time one waits for an examination room and then for the consultation once in it. We said no. He compromised and said he would hurry the test results and meet us in his office the day before we were to leave.

The surgeon had to cancel our appointment with him at his office. It appears that on that day, his furnace went out at home and he had to leave the office to let in the repairmen. We found this comical and I remember wondering what his family members did that a surgeon would be the one to take time off for this task. In fact, the surgeon was very responsible and came to our house at 9 P.M. the evening before we were to leave for New Zealand to tell us the results of the biopsy. I greeted him with the words: "Wait till I tell my friends I have a doctor who made a house call!" He didn't smile. I knew the results then. The rest was just detail.

How I Felt When I Was Given the Diagnosis

The surgeon came to our home to give us my test results since he had to cancel our appointment with him at his office because he had to let the repairmen in to fix his furnace. It was December. We were leaving the next day for a 31-day tour of New Zealand. He passed through our living room full of clothes laid out for our trip, on into the kitchen, and at the table, he went through the state of Michigan booklet explaining cancer, its types, ramifications, and therapies. The booklet used schematic diagrams I was very familiar with. The information contained within it was new, though. He said that the treatment would likely be a four-pronged approach: surgery to remove the cancer, radiation to kill off the surrounding cells, chemotherapy to kill off any drifting cells, and Tamoxifen pills if I turned out to be estrogen receptor positive.

He seemed to want me to get the operation immediately. I remember telling him that I took this very seriously but I was going on this trip as planned first. I wasn't going to ruin my sister's celebration or the vacation my husband and I really needed. When he hesitated, I said if the 31-day vacation interim made that much of a difference, I was going to think very hard about the 2 months I had to wait for the mammogram appointment, the 25-day wait to be retested and whatever scheduling time it was going to take to get me on the operating table. I think that showed him I knew about time commitments and was responsible enough to get help immediately upon our return and not put it off. I was concerned that the cancerous mass would grow that quickly—14 months since my last mammogram and that one showed nothing. He said it was probably growing for about 4 years and was only now detectable.

I knew little about cancer, let alone breast cancer. I wasn't even sure where to get background information. I was deflated but I had a trip to take and a celebration to share. Interestingly, things that would have flustered me during another trip were just shaken off, unimportant, like the owner of a Bed and Breakfast who insinuated herself into our room and wouldn't let us put our luggage on the bed because the bedspread was white. This was insignificant. There were more important things. The cancer was real. There was no getting around that. But it was taking a temporary back seat to our trip and for those 31 days we were going to buck up and have fun enough to last us through the unknown experiences the next 12 months would bring.

My sister had emailed me from time to time during her month in the outback of Australia before we met up with her in New Zealand for our vacation together. In her emails she asked how my mammogram went and I sent newsy emails back to her but didn't mention the mammogram at all, much less the results. This was something I had to tell her and my brother-in-law in person. Twenty-two hours after leaving home we met them as planned in New Zealand. As we settled in the parlor of the B&B in Auckland at about 10 A.M. over a cup of hot chocolate, we told them we had something to tell them about the mammogram. They immediately became serious, listening intently, their faces full of concern as we relayed what we knew to date. We told them I couldn't keep it a secret from them throughout our month together, but my plan was to have the four of us enjoy the trip, not speak of the cancer again, my husband and I to go home, me to have the operation, and count on their help during the radiation and chemotherapy when they got back home from their 3-month vacation a month after us. There wasn't much that I would need their help with until then.

The surgeon and I compromised by having appointments for second opinions 36 hours after we returned from New Zealand. I wondered how they could do that before the operation but did as we'd agreed. None of the medicos examining me could feel the lump. It was the mammogram that found it, and the biopsy that confirmed it.

WHAT MY DOCTOR DID TO HELP ME OVER THE INITIAL SHOCK

My surgeon took over control of my care, scheduling all my appointments, tests, and consultations, answering my questions, etc., from the moment I went in for the confirming mammogram and biopsy. He listened to my concerns. He talked to me. He gave me as much data as he had, which wasn't much. I asked lots of questions. I found there is a frighteningly small amount of statistics out there for breast cancer. Its procedures have progressed steadily, but the long-term data is almost nonexistent.

Early on the surgeon said that I qualified for three different clinical studies and I immediately agreed to participate in two of them. Clearly, they needed data; how else were they going to get it? This was women helping fellow women: basic and essential. Two of the three trials sounded good to me. I signed up for the sentinel node dissection and a blind study that consisted of a California university receiving samples of bone marrow taken during surgery from both my hips to see if they could find something in the marrow that would be an early indicator of cancer. I felt better doing something constructive. I was no longer entirely on the receiving end of medical treatment. Neither procedure caused me any pain—they just required time for follow-up examinations and measurements.

The study I didn't opt into was a random picking of procedure depending on what color ball was chosen. I don't gamble on a normal day and I certainly wasn't going to start with something as important as my health. I wanted to choose, based on the best available knowledge at the time and help expand that base of knowledge in the process.

One of the staff whom the surgeon had me consult with was a social worker who asked me if I felt angry that this was happening to me. I thought that an odd question. Was I unusual? Why did she ask that? Was I supposed to be angry and I wasn't? I felt a lot of things—fear, uncertainty, helplessness—but not anger. After all, the chances are one in eight of getting breast cancer. There were posters all over the surgical area that said breast cancer happens to old and young, heavy and slim, black and white, mothers and childless, smokers and nonsmokers, men and women. Odds are odds. I was just the one that it happened to. I'd only wished that it meant seven others were off the hook. But that's not how statistics work.

How My Family and Friends Reacted to Me and My Disease

That was the most interesting of all the aspects of my cancer. Some people might keep their cancer a secret, telling folks on a need-to-know basis. I'm not that way. I told everyone who would come in close contact with me in the next 12 months. After they were told, we went on with business as usual as much as possible. I knew that my abilities and demeanor were going to fluctuate and I didn't want to hurt folks by saying no or opting out of the projects or declining invitations, not offering to drive, etc., without telling them why. They deserved to know it was me, not them.

My husband, sister, and brother-in-law were my rocks. Not once did my husband say a word, make a grimace, or in any way indicate that he had anything else to do: papers weren't piling up on his desk at work, he wasn't tired or worried or indecisive. He was there for me every minute, supplying smiles, reassurance, and clear logic in an emotional world. When the doctors would schedule yet another visit, he would simply arrange someone to take over the meeting or change the time of it to accommodate me. I was number one in his book. He came to all my consultations so that we had the same two pairs of ears hearing what each doctor said. Then we'd compare notes on what we'd each heard and come up with a more complete understanding of the diagnosis, treatment plan, and prognosis. After each visit to the Henry Ford Hospital Main Campus my husband would take me to Mexicantown for a bite to eat. It was our reward and time to talk to each other about what had just transpired. Celebrating the 1-year anniversary of my first surgery that way was most special. It meant that I'd completed the surgeries, made the decisions, finished the radiation, and started on Tamoxifen without any side effects. I was on my way to that coveted category—Survivorship!

My sister and brother-in-law were there for me, too. I remember one time having the flu so severely I didn't know how I drove the ten miles home from radiation. Though I was feeling better, my sister, whose husband was in a hospital across town at the time insisted on coming over and driving me after she'd seen to her husband earlier in the day. My treatments were at 8:30 A.M., so you can imagine how early in the day she had to check in on her husband before getting to me and how long that made her day. She even built in some time to go shopping. You wouldn't have known there was anything else she had to do all day. We came upon a spectacular sale (1/10 the retail cost) on shirts at Target in my super size, in a yummy yellow shade similar to black-eyed Susans in the sunshine, and so soft on my skin that I bought ten of them! Every time I wear them, I think of the warmth and love and sheer abandon of that day. I felt alive and it was wonderful!

During the entire course of treatments, my closest cousins invited my husband and me over often, sharing birthday parties, Easter, Mothers Day, anything, just to surround me in their love. The food was good too! We'd play cards, watch video movies, talk. It was like being a kid again with no troubles, no worries, no stress.

My method of dealing with the "Big C" was to tell folks. I wanted them to know by my actions and abilities during the treatments, what it was like, and recognize first hand that it wasn't something mysterious — the existence of which should be hidden and hushed. I was neither contagious nor considering a coffin. A fellow volunteer, 85+ years old, drove me to some meetings. "After all, it is a carpool, isn't it?" she said when she learned that my driving required using the driver's side shoulder harness that rubbed across my incision site. Folks I wouldn't have thought were first-string friends jumped in to cheer me and keep my mind off the upcoming procedures, took me to lunch, and generally pampered me. They kept me in the loop of their lives so that I didn't have to dwell on mine. I learned a lot about them in the process. It was a good side effect. They are special people in my life now. I know I can count on them when the chips are down and I make a super effort to be there for them too. They taught me the importance of that.

My neighbor of 30 years, having suffered breast cancer 10 years before, delayed her winter sojourn to Florida until I was home from the hospital safe and sound. I remember sitting at my exercise machine doing my leg exercises, anything to keep moving, and telling her I was Stage 1, T1, invasive ductal, estrogen receptor positive and saying, "Do you know what those things mean?"

and her saying, "Yes, I know all of it." In her soothing way, she said to think of this as just a bump in the road of life and that I would be fine. I said, "Do you mind if I call you in Florida sometimes just to talk?" She told me I could call her as often as I wished and whenever I wished for any reason at all. I never felt closer to her than at that moment.

A day or two after my first lumpectomy, another friend who'd had cancer called and invited herself over. She arrived bearing a tray of marvelous homemade minimuffins. We put on water for tea and she told me what was upcoming and what to expect. She was a survivor. Like a big sister, she was there to lead me through the rough parts so I wouldn't be overwhelmed. I never knew that take-charge side of her before. That was when I realized I'd joined a special club of cancer carriers. They were there for me. And I, too, could be a survivor!

I was one who needed the support of family and friends and got it. I kept up with some folks via email and kept the correspondences in a computer folder, not deleting any, so that I could go through them when I felt drained or depressed. I never had to open that folder. Family and friends kept up the concern for the length of my therapy. It was wonderful. Email helped. People I didn't know had cancer shared their experiences with me. It was only my mentioning mine that brought it to the fore. I didn't blab it around, but I did mention a line or two to folks who asked how I was so that they knew the procedures I was undergoing and therefore how cancer could get "fixed." Some, like myself, hadn't previously had a clue. We were learning together.

So many things came into perspective during that year. Not only did I learn a lot about the body and cancer but I taught folks about it too and came to new understandings, for instance, why my minimuffin-toting-chemo-taking friend called me at a volunteers meeting that was already underway and everyone who was going to be there was in attendance. She asked if anyone had a cold or was coughing before she decided it was safe to come over. Undergoing chemo, her immune system was compromised and she couldn't afford to take the chance on catching a bug, but she did so want to come to the meeting of her friends. I assured her "the coast was clear." She came to the meeting and we all had a great time together.

Was everyone nurturing and helpful and hopeful and uplifting during my course of cancer treatment? Of course not. Some distanced themselves. I could tell by the way they looked at me when they asked how I was that they didn't really want an answer. Their body language confirmed this. So I'd just say, "I'm doing well," which was true. Thank goodness I didn't need them. One said to call her to go out to lunch when I wanted somebody who wouldn't mention cancer in any way. She seemed to think that I would be so totally absorbed in the subject that I'd be unable to think or talk about anything else and I would appreciate the respite. She was wrong. Cancer didn't rule my life. On the other hand, not talking about it didn't make it go away. It was the interaction with family and friends and their lives and happenings that brought me through. I preferred to briefly mention the status of my cancer, and then move on to something interesting in their lives. In fact, during the course of my treatments, while awaiting doctors' consultations, I crocheted two wedding afghans for cousins. A brother and sister were getting married seven weeks apart, beginning 2 months after I finished radiation. Other patients and caregivers and staff would stop and comment on the colors or pattern and we'd chat about the upcoming weddings and similar happenings in their families. Nothing was said about cancer, nor did it need to be. We were celebrating life together.

THE SURGICAL OPERATION

The surgical operation was going to answer some questions. It was also Step 1 of my therapy to get rid of this *weed* in the *native perennial garden* I call my body. I wanted it removed out as quickly as possible.

It was party time in pre-op. The nurses and staff were upbeat and friendly and concerned. With the interest of a medical student, I took three injections of technetium-99 (the radioactive element with a half life of 6 hours) to mark the sentinel node. Fortunately, the blue dye injected into me drained to the same node as the one the radioactive element found by the gamma probe so there was good probability that was the sentinel node and would be the first one the cancer cells would also drain into. When I woke up from the anesthesia, they'd taken out that sentinel node only and a 1.3 cm cancerous mass. That was the good news. I came home and emailed everybody!

The bad news came a few days later: there were minute traces of cancer cells in the "margins"—the edges of the lump they removed. Not knowing for sure whether it was the tail end of a tentacle or a line to another primary site, I underwent a second surgery 10 days later where the surgeon took out another centimeter slice and it showed clean margins. Hurray! There was pretty good certainty they'd gotten it all—unless it traveled to another part of my body or skipped the sentinel node. Always some bit of uncertainty. But then I could walk out in the street and get run over by a truck. Life is uncertain. My husband was in the waiting room and that thought made me feel better. He was there, ready to take me home, when I came to consciousness again.

RADIATION

I'm claustrophobic and have a bad back. Getting spotted for radiation didn't sound like fun to me. "Lie still and don't move for 45 minutes on this hard table so we can mark the spots used to focus on the areas we are going to radiate" could have been a problem. To help ease my jumpy nerves, I asked them to tell me what they would be doing and where in that list we were as we went along and to please not leave me there while going out for a coffee break or lunch or to take a phone call or do another consult. Moving efficiently, making me as comfortable as possible, all the while saying I was doing fine, they completed the marking task without incident. My doctor was new to this hospital and its staff, yet she and they worked together as a team getting the job done quickly and correctly. The success of the marking procedure eased my concerns. The actual radiation treatments were quick and painless.

I drew a regular schedule of 34 sessions of radiation and come hell or high water I was going to be there for every one of them, having to be driven twice during the program because flu made me too woozy to drive myself. That was a nice thing about radiation. It was independent of my other health problems. As long as I could get my body there, I could receive treatment. I called the radiation machine Steely Dan because its ID plate, which was pretty much in my face when the machine was in position to radiate me, said it was made of steel, and I hummed in time to its sounds while I was in there. It was comfortable, didn't hurt, and the technicians and office staff were great. We became friends and I gave them a CD of Steely Dan music as a thank-you gift for being so consistently nice and efficient and professional with me. It wasn't until I was three quarters of the way through my regimen that I found out the two technologists were brother and sister. I don't see resemblances in twins much less siblings so I was happy they told me. I thought they worked really well together and they treated me like I was part of their family.

During the course of radiation treatment, I came to know the patients in the waiting room. One whose appointment was just before mine had seven sites of cancer in 9 years, and they were treating her brain at the moment. She'd lost her job over the amount of time she'd missed work and so did her caregiver brother due to downsizing. He'd bring her in and dote like you'd expect a big brother to do. She'd be coming out of the radiation room as I was going in and she would say she'd warmed up the table and machine for me. I in turn passed that on to the patient following me. On her last day, near Easter, I presented her with a cute cuddly stuffed bunny with long ears to remember our times together. I often wonder how she is faring, and I send a little positive thought out to her.

The patient after me was a fellow who had prostate cancer, and his wife would wait for him to go into the radiation room and then go to the coffee kiosk and get him a great big latte, a treat he loved. Looking at all these brave people receiving radiation and wonderful staff who facilitated it, I knew I was probably the healthiest person they'd see all day. To make them smile and brighten their day a bit was the least I could do. It wasn't hard. They were my cancer family.

CHEMOTHERAPY

The surgeon who'd set up my treatment plan had groomed me to expect chemo as the second of four prongs to recovery: surgery, chemo, radiation, and Tamoxifen if I was found to be estrogen receptor positive. When the oncologist surprisingly and abruptly dismissed himself from my case, I was left standing in an empty field. I felt I had failed some test. What did I do to make him feel there was no recourse but to eliminate me from his practice?

He wouldn't tell me. Was I that bad with the other doctors too? The protocol was to hand me from specialist to specialist. The surgeon had signed off on me and I was in the hands of the oncologist who'd just divorced me. Now what?

I had to find a new doctor and start over. Leftover from the first doctor was the prospect of getting a port put in since my only good vein was in the same arm that was on that side of my body that could no longer get compromised in any way. The port would be a ball under my skin that had a silicone catheter connecting it to a vein deep in my body. Whatever was injected into the ball found its way into that vein and whatever was withdrawn (blood for testing) was taken out of the vein via that ball. They gave me the phone number and I had to make my own appointment and arrangements. Meanwhile, the appointment with the new oncologist was to be 2 days after I was to get the port put in. I got to thinking about it and decided it wasn't fair for the new doctor to follow a regimen set up by the first doctor. He might have his own theories and I wanted to hear them before undergoing more surgery. I left a message asking him to give me a quick call, which he actually did at 7:15 on a Friday night from the hospital. My first thought was "Wow, this guy is really dedicated." He asked me not to put in the port until I talked to him. When my husband and I walked into his office, his first question was if I'd put in the port. I said no. He said, "Good, have a seat and let's talk."

An hour later, he'd explained to us another possibility, saying the dangers of chemo outweighed the advantages in my case. He was giving me options, not emotions, and treating me like a thinking, analyzing, adult, fellow human being. He said, "Well you have one yes, do chemo, and one no, don't. I suppose you'd like to have a third opinion." He'd read my mind. Further, he told me that whatever I decided, he'd be proud to be my doctor. I was elated! After having been dismissed by the first chemo doctor, here was one who also got to know me and would be happy to take me on, no matter which road I chose. I felt worthy again. He then called in the social worker and together they found a way to get me that third opinion. Chemo Doctor 3 said that the pendulum swings for chemo for a few years and then against it and right now it was for it. Great! One yes, one no, one maybe.

It was becoming clear that I'd be the one to say yea or nay to chemo. We'd met some cousins for breakfast and I caught up with their lives but didn't mention the intrusion of cancer into mine. After we said goodbye to the cousins we climbed into my sister's minivan and talked. My husband, sister, and brother-in-law gave me the pros and cons as they saw it, but didn't tell me what to do. I wouldn't ask them to, either. That wouldn't be fair to them. It was my body and my responsibility. If anything went wrong, there would be no guilt for anyone else.

One thing the second chemo doctor said kept coming to mind: chemo attacked all the fast growing cells, not just the cancer cells. Everyone knew about the loss of hair and nails, but chemo also compromised the heart, lungs, liver, and could cause blood clots, which were pretty serious. So one could conceivably cause more harm than good in getting the chemo done than doing without it. And the chemo in my case only raised my odds 1–2 percent. If I wanted to increase my odds that amount, he said, I should eat healthy, not drink or smoke, think happy thoughts, lose some weight, exercise regularly, and reduce stress. I thought a lot about it. It was hard, but I decided against taking chemo. Sure, I was afraid of the effects of the drugs every 3 weeks, but choosing not to do chemo was in direct conflict with my mindset since day 1 when the surgeon said my treatment included chemotherapy. If I didn't do it, was I somehow deviating from the regimen as planned? Was I shirking my duty to myself? Was I compromising my health because I didn't want to spend the next 6 months upchucking? Or was it the right thing to do? I had to force myself to make a logical decision, overcoming mindsets and emotions. The chemo doctor went on to say that even though I was postmenopausal, Tamoxifen pills could be taken daily for 5 years since my cancer tested estrogen receptor positive, meaning the estrogen in my body was the catalyst for the cancer cell growth. Killing all the estrogen in my body would slowly starve the cancer cells if there were any floating around. That made sense too. Soymilk was out too, since soy helps produce estrogen. Now it's rice milk for this lactose intolerant cancer survivor-to-be! Amazing what you can get used to.

The first chemo doctor had actually done me a great favor. His actions allowed me to meet and be treated by a new doctor in whom I have full confidence and comfort, and pursue a different course of action entirely, one that made sense to me. Time will tell if I chose wisely.

How I Was Able/Not Able to Work during My Treatment

I do contract work and volunteer work that could be done when I was home and in good stead. These things, far from tiring me, kept me thinking of other things and people. I thought that I had everything under control and was keeping up with things. Then, one day, I looked in the medicine cabinet for the cough syrup and realized it had expired 2 years before. The same applied to the food supplies in the basement and salad dressings in the refrigerator. I guess some things did escape me after all. But the important things—connections with family and friends and treatments—were under control. That's what counted.

My Spiritual Connection

This doesn't take the form of prayer wheels, novenas, and lighted candles, but it is definitely spiritual in that I learned a lot about how the body is made, how cells reproduce, how they automatically correct themselves from going awry, and how intricately and complicatedly and beautifully we are made by the Creator of All Things. That knowledge is awesome and I might never have explored it to the extend I did if I didn't delve into what was happening with my own body. When I was in for presurgical second opinions, one of the "stations" I visited was with a lady who had had cancer and was there to answer practical questions and to console me. She kept asking me if I wanted to pray with her. I kept saying I had questions that I'd feel better if I had answers to since I had some important decisions to make. At that moment I needed knowledge, data, statistics and percentages. I'm an engineer. This is how I tackle a problem and make a determination. It is also where I look for and find God. That is my connection. Some say the devil is in the details. I think sometimes God is.

MY BIGGEST FEAR

Parting from my loved ones was my greatest fear. I was surrounded by love, but the decisions were mine alone to make and if I chose incorrectly, it might be exactly what would part me from them. It was physically hard to breathe sometimes with that weight on my chest.

MY MOST MEMORABLE EXPERIENCE

Coming out of lumpectomy surgery the first time was like a party, with folks talking loud to me to get me out of the anesthetic and offering me painkillers and juice and graham crackers (my comfort food to this day). People were everywhere: fellow patients, nurses, orderlies, caregivers. I had to have two lumpectomies since the first lump they removed had traces of cancer in the margins.

The second event was very different. I slowly awoke from surgery, alone, in a private room with a constant buzzing going on behind my head. I couldn't move my arms or legs without concerted effort and even then not very far. No one was around. I thought the buzzing was one of those machines indicating a flat line on breathing or heart rate like they show on TV. I concluded I'd died. Then a nurse came in and shut off the buzzer and offered me the juice and graham crackers (love those graham crackers). The buzzer was from the oxygen sensor coming loose on my finger. That answered question one. I was alive. But why the private room? Did something go wrong during the surgery? No, she said. They take us to whatever bed is available. Boy was I relieved! But I missed the bustle.

Every time someone asks me how I am doing I get this huge smile on my face and say, "Just fine. Thanks for asking!" and mean it. Every day is a blessing.

When I had my last 6-month maintenance visit before starting on a once-a-year plan, my chemo doctor said, "Get out of my office and make room for someone who is sick." What an insightful sense of humor he has. I smile every time I think of it! I was only too happy to oblige him! The message was that I'm not sick anymore but could come back if I needed to. He'd certainly be there for me.

MY ADVICE TO WOMEN WITH NEWLY DIAGNOSED
BREAST CANCER

Get the facts. Listen to emotional rhetoric and people's anecdotal experiences, if you like. But you can't possibly talk to everybody about cancer so you must know the statistics if you are to make an informed decision.

Participate actively in your treatment plan. You are going to have to make hard decisions. Others can advise you but you are wisest to take control of your own treatment. I was thrust into that position when my first chemo doctor divorced himself from my case and that turned out to be the best thing he could have done for me. It brought me into contact with another doctor who had more information and with whom I had confidence and I made a different, more informed decision subsequently due to it. I have every reason to believe it is the right one for me, based on the results of tests so far.

Some have said a good attitude won't cure cancer. That is true. But an optimistic attitude will help others be able to approach you and give of themselves emotionally without being overwhelmed themselves. They're saying, "We're there for you if you'll let us lift you up and you not drag us down." Their support can't be understated. Make your mindset such that you are able to be lifted up and then let them do it. You'll feel better and so will they.

Reach out. Teach others by your actions that cancer isn't the end of the world. They probably know very little about the disease and a sentence or two on what it is or your treatment plan and where you are in it at the moment helps a lot of people understand the whole disease. "Did you know that cells reproduce themselves often and that the body has several ways to monitor the cells and correct them before they get too far afield? Cancer cells somehow slip by unchecked. Medicos don't know why. But it is that simple and yet that complicated." This teaches as well as assures folks that it's just something that happens. "Cancer is only a bump in the road of life," as my neighbor said. And it can be cured in a lot of cases!

Do not let the cancer destroy your sense of self. You are who you are regardless of the size and/or shape of your breasts or the presence of other body parts. Looking as good as you can look should always take a back seat to being as good as you can! You're a total person, no matter what your front looks like or how many body parts you are missing. And anybody who tells you otherwise is missing your best part—your personality!

Participate in everything you can, including medical trials and clinical studies, which will give the medical community more information and statistics. They can't do this without us. In its own way, this is more important than monetary donations. Hard data is our legacy to the next generation.

This experience is gaining you a lot of knowledge about yourself, others, life, and what matters. Learn from it. Gain depth. Be there for others who have cancer or any other problem you might be able to help with. We need each other.

I was fortunate that I had family and friends I could count on. Now it's my turn to be the family and friend others can count on. That's my payback.

Get involved with a project that will last the length of time of your treatment. When your treatments are finished so are your projects. I crocheted two afghans for cousins getting married and grew my hair out so I could donate ten 13-inch ponytails of thick dark naturally curly hair to an organization called Locks of Love. They use donations to make natural hair wigs for children who have lost their hair due to alopecia or leukemia. I met little Heather while getting my hair cut during a promotion at city hall and my heart went out to her. She'd just gotten fitted with a wig. I told the stylist to cut off as much of my hair as she possibly could to be able to give the little ones as much length as possible. She said I had so much hair they could probably make a whole wig of my hair alone. I was delighted to share. During the 20 months it took to grow my hair that long, I was a walking billboard, telling folks why I was doing it. They deserved to know since a 56-year-old in pigtails needed some explaining. I got about five people to donate their hair too. This is something constructive we could do to help our little sisters.

Get your mammograms on whatever regular basis your doctor sets up for you. No one ever felt my lump. I call the mammogram machine the "jaws of life."

MISCELLANEOUS

I took my radiation treatments at SJHS in Clinton Township. The cancer center there has a huge tank with lovely and unique tropical fish and an information card to describe each of them. They seemed to get fed on a regular regimen and I gauged my progress through radiation based on their feeding. It was an internal time clock shared with these lovely creatures. I wasn't satisfied until I'd found each of them in their hiding spaces. It was a daily game of hide and seek we played with each other.

The radiation receptionist was a big fan of giraffes. She had them on in some form almost every day: earrings, shirt appliqué, bracelet, picture on her desk. She was so sweet and we'd discuss giraffes. It became a game like finding Kilroy in a picture. She's long since retired but, to this day, I can't see a giraffe and not think of her smiling face and her pleasant and peaceful disposition.

Pamela Brady impresses us with her *humanity*—her obvious love of life and other people, her willingness to share her experience and what she learned from it, and her generosity.

Because of her intelligence and observational powers she learned from her experiences. Her story is important because it mirrors the main messages of the book. These are helpful lessons from someone who has already experienced a major change in her own life.

If you were to mention Pamela's courage to her, I suspect she would get a puzzled expression on her face. Her courage, like many people's, is simply a quiet part of her character as she faces whatever challenges that life sends her way.

As you read her "case study," you probably saw other aspects of Pamela's experience and made comparisons with your own situation—either what you are immersed in or what you are anticipating. Not everyone can see breast cancer as just "a bump in the road of life." But I believe that most people are capable of the kind of inner strength that Pamela Brady showed us. I know this from my 40 years of experience in treating breast cancer patients, and I know it from the stories that make up the rest of this book. The following chapters highlight the variety of women's experiences with breast cancer.

We begin with a look at how they first detected their cancers.

2

DETECTION: "IT WAS A NICE SPRING DAY . . ."

Early detection of breast cancer is a crucial factor in the successful "miracle" of recovery. The stories told by cancer survivors demonstrate that the disease was usually first detected either by an abnormal finding on routine mammogram or feeling a lump, but there were a variety of responses to the discovery. These responses are important because, as most patients know and more and more doctors are realizing, treatment of cancer is in reality the treatment of the patient, the human being, and not just the treatment of the cells that are growing within the body of the human being. The feelings, emotions, and experiences of the person become a natural part of the treatment and recovery process.

Several of the women responding to our questionnaire were brief and matter-of-fact in describing the discovery of their breast cancer. Bettie said, "I found a lump in my right breast," and Gwendolyn simply said, "Mammogram." In fact, mammograms were crucial first steps toward treatment for many, as Margaret reports: "Discovered through my regular mammogram—never skip this important exam, NEVER!" Lisa tells a similar story: "I'm one of the increasing number of lucky ones. The small lump in my right breast was detected by a routine mammogram and follow-up." Ethel, like many of the women who reported, was surprised by her mammogram results: "My breast cancer was discovered during a routine mammogram when I was 78. I was surprised because I felt so good physically and there was no family history of breast cancer but I did not feel shocked or frightened. My family and friends were supportive and positive, and Dr. Nathanson's approach helped to put me at ease."

Routine mammograms were not the only first steps. Sally Cole-Saul's alertness helped her detect her first breast cancer: "My first instance of breast cancer occurred in 1993; I was on a cruise ship with my mom. We were doing a dance for the passenger show when I was accidentally hit in the right breast. It hurt and I could feel a very small lump. The first biopsy was inconclusive. I insisted on having the lump removed (about 4–5 mm), and the subsequent pathology indicated that it was cancer. My second instance occurred in 1998. A lump was seen in the mammogram in my left breast. It was also positive for cancer (although a different kind of cancer)." Marianne also discovered the lump by herself: "Palpating my breasts, I discovered it and asked the ultrasound technician to pay special attention to where I was pointing," and Jeanette said, "My primary doctor felt the small lump in my breast. I had the biopsy and was scheduled for surgery." Jackie was the only woman who reported her husband's finding the lump: "I always had my regular mammograms. I had one 3 months prior to my husband finding the lump on my left breast."

I suspect that the emotions these women expressed may have been so low-key because of the item-by-item format of the questionnaire. The passage of time may also have caused some of the emotions to fade.

Shock was a more common response to detection. Hardeep said starkly, "I felt as if I were given a Death Sentence. As if I were in a nightmare, if I would go to sleep it might go away when I woke up." In the following account, Roxanne continues in that tone of voice: "I found the tumor! One evening, I was watching a program on TV and felt a shooting pain. It was so hard I jumped! And my first reaction was to reach my left breast with my right hand and you don't want to know the words that came out of my mouth. I felt the lump. Immediately, I felt a feeling of terror that invaded my whole body. I didn't say anything to anyone and 2 weeks later, I called and tried to set up an appointment with my gynecologist. I really didn't know who to go to. I considered the problem as a 'female problem.' That was Dr. R. He examined me, wished me good luck and gave me the referral to the surgeon. There was not much he could say."

The "feeling of terror" is an entirely natural response, as is some initial confusion about which doctor to see—where to start the process of treatment and recovery.

Many breast cancer patients are not totally surprised by the discovery of a lump, either because of a family history of breast cancer or the discovery of lumps in the past. Understanding the possibility of breast cancer does not always shield a person from shock, as Becky's account shows:

"My breast cancer journey starts with the death of my 33-year-old niece Dawn, diagnosed at age 25. I was diagnosed 1 month later at age 45, September 2001. My cancer was discovered through a routine mammogram. They found suspicious microcalcifications. My biopsy was on September 11, a sad day for a lot of people and one I will never forget. My doctor called me that Thursday telling me to come in and discuss my new found cancer. I was sick and frightened, for I had just seen my niece die from this horrid disease, expecting the same for myself." The words "frightened" and "horrid" reflect emotions shared by many women in that situation. Here the horror of cancer is associated with the horror of September 11.

Francine made a similar association with that tragedy:

"It's November of 2001 and everyone is still quite on the edge after the terrorists attacks of 9-11. I went in to HFH for my yearly physical. My primary care physician detected a lump in my left breast and wanted it further checked at the Breast Clinic. I made the appointment for late in the month and tried not to worry since I had had a recheck years ago and it was just calcifications. But always in the back of my mind was the thought that my mother had breast cancer at a similar age. At my breast clinic appointment Dr. Nathanson examined me and sent me for a mammogram. I was then sent for an ultrasound and biopsy . . . by now I'm really getting anxious. I'm sent home and told to come back in about a week for results. The only person I share this with is my husband."

Often the experience of waiting—for appointments or for biopsy results—intensifies the fear and anxiety. While you are waiting you feel like you are doing nothing to gain an understanding and begin treatment.

In Sally W.'s account of her life-changing discovery, we see how she turned both her panic and the horrible weather into a solution to the anxiety of waiting:

"On New Year's Eve in 1999 we didn't venture out. The weather was calling for more snow and slippery conditions. A quiet evening at home with a few glasses of wine with crackers and cheese and a good movie sounded fine to us. We were getting ready for bed and I was just finishing my shower. I did a breast exam as I do every time I think about it. Just to be sure I repeated the steps while I was lying down in bed. Clockwise and counterclockwise with my fingertips as I extended the arm on the same side I was examining. I froze with fear not wanting to believe I was feeling something that shouldn't be there. I kept my finger on the spot and asked my husband if he could feel it. He said he felt a small hard bump about the size of a small pea.

"I was glad Monday was only a few days away and I had a scheduled appointment with internal medicine. The snow was pretty deep and we were expecting more. That actually turned out to be the only lucky turn of events for the next few weeks. Dr. V., my regular doctor, was out of town so I was scheduled to see Dr. D. I told him about my lump. He checked me and sent me down for a mammogram appointment. He also wrote an order for an ultrasound. I went down to x-ray to make my appointment and found I could get right in for my mammogram. People were not showing up for their scheduled appointments because of the weather. The doctor who read the mammogram was very sympathetic to my fragile emotional state. She knew something was not normal on the x-ray and left the room for a moment. When she came back into the room she told me I could have my ultrasound next. I was so glad I could get these things done so quickly. I didn't want any time to dwell on things. After the ultrasound, the doctor said I needed to have a biopsy done and the nurse would make the appointment with Dr. Nathanson. I was scared and upset and just waiting to hear that awful 'C' word. When can I see the doctor? He is very busy; it may take a few weeks. The nurse saw the panic in my eyes and left the room to make the phone call. My mind was racing. I would surely lose my mind in less than a few weeks, I thought, making myself dizzy with the thought. When the nurse came back she said my appointment would be in 3 days and he would do the biopsy at the same time. What a nurse."

Somehow people find a way to get through the experience. If the cancer is a terrible accident, then the weather and the encounter with an alert and compassionate nurse are happy accidents. Training health care professionals to respond constructively to their patients' emotional needs is not at all accidental.

Many women are aware of the possibility of breast cancer because of their personal or family history. This awareness encourages early detection, but it does not eliminate the feeling of shock and surprise, as Beverly's account shows:

"My journey with cancer started in my 72nd year with a visit to my dermatologist who has been treating me for skin cancer for years. On a visit to his office the inquiry of how are you feeling prompted, 'I'm so tired.' He recommended a physical, so I made an appointment with Dr. M., my husband's internist.

"Dr. M. was very thorough and the mammogram showed a lump in my left breast. I was not too concerned as I had surgery on my right breast in 1978 with the results of a cyst—but this time the six biopsies ordered showed cancer."

Like Beverly, Judith was surprised at the discovery of a lump, even though her personal history made her aware of the possibility of breast cancer:

"I have had fibrocystic breast disease since the late 1970s and had several lumps aspirated over the years, which were benign. They watched me closely after I went on hormone therapy in 1990 because of my past history, and I had had no problems.

"However, I discovered the lump that was cancerous in my left breast along the breast bone during my monthly self breast exam in early August of 2001. I had my yearly mammogram in December of 2000 in Kalamazoo, and they saw nothing suspicious. So I was really surprised to find this lump in early August. Although, when I look back on my records, my internist did say there was a thickening at that spot when I had my physical in November of 2000, but I didn't think anything about it nor did he. Because of where it was located, the mammograms didn't detect the lump that close to the center of the chest."

The vigilance that is so important to early detection and treatment does not mitigate the feelings of surprise and shock.

We are all reluctant to accept bad news, or even the possibility of bad news, as in Alyce's response to her discovery:

"It was a hot day in July. I had just been dismissed from the hospital, where I'd had minor surgery and as I walked into my apartment the phone was ringing. It was my internist who told me the mammogram I'd had was suspicious and he wanted me to see a surgeon. I assured him every time I had a mammogram I was given the same report. However, I agreed to go."

Moving beyond shock and denial to acceptance is an important step. Julia described a similar move:

"I was totally shocked at the breast cancer found. I had gone for a physical examination, feeling great, so I figured I was fine and the physical would confirm it. Each step after the first diagnosis, I believed that it would be all a big mistake, yet a part of me said be realistic, they don't come up with these determinations without plenty of evidence. So I accepted it reluctantly."

Her reluctance, of course, is totally normal. Julia went on to say, "When hit with cancer suddenly, you realize how carefully you have brainwashed yourself to believe that it will never get you." Julia's resilience is evident in her moving through denial ("all a big mistake") to a rational understanding.

Moving past shock and denial to acceptance and an active and engaged attitude is very important emotionally. Note how Clara made an important emotional shift when she explained the likely cause of her cancer:

"I had just finished bathing and was using astringent, before oil, on my legs. As I bent over, my right breast burned as it touched my leg. I was alarmed and looked at my breast: the nipple was diminished and raw, but not oozing any liquid. I was scared, and decided to call Fairlane Henry Ford H.S. to get a biopsy. They told me I'd have to call Henry Ford Hospital, so I did, and made an appointment to have a biopsy with the dermatologist. I also had three small growths on my face. The one on my right side of my chin was like a bubble and bled. It and my breast nipple were positive for cancer. They called the one on my breast nipple and milk ducts 'Paget's disease.'

"The dermatologist was very patient, kind, and careful as could be, but when she put the needle with Novocaine in my nipple, my feet almost hit the ceiling. I didn't yell but it hurt so bad I lost control. That was to deaden the nerve so she could take a biopsy.

"I must explain how this originated, but at the time I didn't realize it was going to cause cancer: I was a hairdresser and I had a 2-year-old sitting in my chair. Just as I was about to cut he turned his head, and the scissors went into my hand. I was sent to the clinic to be stitched. They gave me a tetanus shot and a prescription for antibiotics. I told them I had had reactions from antibiotics twice. He said, 'This shouldn't cause any; it's a generic made for people with allergies.' So I took it, and when I had only one capsule left my breast bled. I called the doctor at the clinic. He said to stop taking it. I threw the last one away and in a couple of days everything was OK. I didn't have any pain or stomach trouble, so I thought everything is normal. But then I started getting brown spots on my skin all over my body.

"I called Fairlane HFH Clinic and made an appointment to have a complete physical. They took a cholesterol blood check. It came back very high. I was given a lean heart health smart diet. They told me the brown marks were from coffee and sun. So I quit coffee, got a big hat, covered up and used 30–40 sunblock. I went to Fairlane HFH Clinic to see if I could get more blood tests taken. They said I had to get a doctor's order. (The brown spots were increasing and I was getting fatigue.) I made an appointment with the doctor. They both, the doctor and the nurse, thought I was a hypochondriac. The nurse said, 'Just what are you doing here?' I told her the spots were increasing and now I was getting fatigue. The reason they didn't think anything was wrong with me was because I was in excellent physical condition, so I looked healthy. I was very active all my life and did exercises. Because of allergies, I had to. That was my last doctor's visit."

As with many cancer patients, Clara's ability to *understand* gave her some sense of control, even though it did not lead to a cure. Understanding—even partial understanding—lifts people from helplessness toward resilience and recovery.

We see a striking example of the turn from despair toward resiliency in Linda's story:

"I am a health care worker. In fact, I am an x-ray technologist with a subspecialty in mammography. I scheduled myself for my routine mammogram at the facility where I work. By coincidence, I happened to be working in the mammography section the morning of my exam. After my exam had been completed by my coworker, I remember looking at the developed films thinking that there was a serious problem for someone. That 'someone' turned out to be me. Those were my films! When I left work that day, although I had not been officially diagnosed, I knew in my heart that I had breast cancer.

"I remember lying in bed that first night thinking, 'Cancer. I'm going to die. Well, maybe if I don't close my eyes, I won't die.' So, consequently, I lay there all night not daring to close my eyes for fear I would not wake up. When the sun shone the next day, I knew that no matter what the outcome of my disease, I certainly wasn't going to die that day!"

Linda's recovery began with the resilience shown in her concluding realization.

An important feature of resilience for many women is their ability to see humor in even the gravest of situations. D'Anna described her discovery as follows:

"I was walking up stairs on Sunday evening after Thanksgiving in 1999, when I felt a sharp pain in my right breast. I reached up with my left hand and discovered a lump. Whoa, where did that come from? I had had a clean mammogram in February of that year. I had an appointment with my PCP for a pap smear in about 3 weeks, and I debated whether to wait until then or try to get in earlier. By Monday afternoon, I had called and scheduled an earlier appointment.

"My doctor didn't think that it was anything to be concerned about, but she wanted me to have a mammogram. She suggested the name of a surgeon, but I asked if I could see Dr. Nathanson. I knew of three people who had seen him for breast cancer, and I also knew him from working in the lab next door to his at Henry Ford Hospital.

"After the mammogram I was told to schedule an appointment for an ultrasound. Stupid me, I didn't know what this meant, so I made an appointment. At the ultrasound, the doctor wanted to do a core needle biopsy. I was totally unprepared for this, but I figured they might as well do it. They attempted to numb the area, but after the first biopsy I was almost passing out from the pain.

They lowered the head of the bed and injected more numbing agent before they continued with the biopsies. They were all painful, but I got through the rest and returned to work. I went home that night and told my husband they had poked holes in me!"

We can sense that humor is deeply engrained in D'Anna's character, and I suspect that she may have even seen the humor a few short hours after her painful experience.

Others get through the shock of discovery thanks to an optimistic attitude that they carry with them. Listen to Beatrice's tone of voice:

"It's hard to revisit the cancer days not because it was unpleasant but rather because there's so much to relate and it's hard to say it honestly. It started on August 17, 2001, my mother and dad's anniversary . . . both gone many years. But it was a well-known date, one of celebration that we managed to share often.

"On that date I had a mammogram. As soon as the mammographer asked me to stay for a more specific set of pictures, I knew they'd find a tumor tucked in among the scar tissue from previous benign biopsies. How did I know? My life is a happy one. I am retired from work that I enjoyed, to join my husband in his retirement. Our daughters and their families live within 10–20 minutes of our home. We have other dear family and friends, some from childhood and others from many close relationships within 50+ years of marriage.

"I am an optimist and have few fears. At 74 years, many diseases and accidents have visited friends and family. Actually, breast cancer has been a part of most women's lives. In any gathering there are breast cancer patients, or survivors, or connections with those from family or friends who have had it. It is not a question of *if*, but of *when*."

We see a similar optimism and confidence in Heidi's account:

"On December 28, 2002, I was scheduled for my annual mammogram. On January 3, 2003, I was contacted by telephone informing me that additional imaging studies were required. On January 6, 2003, I returned to the clinic for another mammogram and ultrasound, which showed a suspicious abnormality. Further testing was suggested and I was scheduled for a mammotome biopsy at the Main Campus. The result was a ductal carcinoma in situ.

"Having experienced invasive breast cancer in 1990, followed by a mastectomy of my right breast and having been informed that a ductal carcinoma in situ means a noninvasive cancer, I accepted this condition, remained calm and positive, and was confident that my medical team would find the best solution to treat me."

I am struck by the calm acceptance in both stories. Heidi was not surprised. I suspect that the optimistic attitudes of both women were important to their recoveries.

Linda P., another patient, became more than frightened when she learned of her cancer. Note how she made an emotional turn:

"It was a nice spring day in April of 2000. I had an appointment for my annual physical with its tests, labs, and of course a mammogram. My doctor found nothing unusual during the exam but something was picked up on the mammogram. I wasn't especially concerned when I was called for a redo of the mammogram as I've had fatty cysts in the past, but I was suspicious when I was sent to the main campus for an ultrasound. It was at that time the cancer was found and when two doctors came out to talk to me I just knew the news wasn't good. In fact, I became hysterical and could only think I was going to die. Thank goodness my husband was with me and the doctors were comforting as they could be but I didn't hear anything except the 'Big C.' You really need a couple of days for the news to sink in so you can rethink your options and talk to your doctors intelligently."

Her becoming hysterical at the news is no surprise. Important in her account is the emotional support from her husband and the doctors, and the fact that after a couple of days the emotion had spent itself, the news had sunk in, and she was able to rethink her options and talk to her doctors intelligently. This is typical of the emotional resilience I have seen time and again.

Detection was followed by diagnosis. While for many women the detection of a lump in the breast does not mean breast cancer, for those in this book the result is not a happy one. On the other hand, the diagnosis is not really the result—in the sense of the final conclusion. It is more like the beginning of the "ordinary miracle" of their recovery.

3

Diagnosis: "This Can't Be Happening to Me"

Receiving news of the actual diagnosis of breast cancer evokes much of the same shock and fear we saw with the detection stories in the previous chapter. Most of the fears that women described occurred immediately after diagnosis.

Lisa spoke for many: "*This can't be happening to me* was my first reaction to the diagnosis of breast cancer." She added. "My husband was recovering from the Moh procedure for recently diagnosed skin cancer. My concerns were for his care." Bettie said simply, "It felt a little scary," and Toni said, "Nausea." Marianne's emotions were at a similar place: "I felt miserable, crying. I had gone for my annual mammogram *alone* and was given the news . . . I was afraid of dying and not being able to be with my family that is very far from where I am." Again and again, women reported the same responses to the diagnosis, with Hardeep saying, "When I first got the call from Dr. D. regarding the results of the mammogram, I was so shocked, I could not even speak to him, I had to hand the phone to my husband to make the further appointments, etc." And Gwen stated, "I was afraid and I thought I would die. My biggest fears were chemotherapy and death." Similarly for Margaret: "My biggest fear was complete mastectomy, which did *not have* to happen—or inability to be cured."

For some, such as Roxanne her fears and anxieties extended into the social context in which she works:

"Finally, I had my mammogram. The doctor that checked it had a worried look on her face. When I finally met with the surgeon and he gave me the news, I felt a sense of helplessness, I felt so alone in this world, I was not afraid to die, but for some reason (I guess due to the terror of hearing what you already know), I was hearing it out loud, 'We found the tumor to be cancerous.' I was angry, sad, and lonely. I wanted to die. Now, I had to tell them at work! I worked with all men! Oh Lord, please I don't want to do this!! I did it. It was not easy."

Her "I did it" was a crucial step for her.

Francine's concerns took a similar turn to considering the impact on other people:

"When I return I am told that I have cancer. It feels like someone punched me in the stomach! I am given my options—I choose the sentinel node biopsy and lumpectomy and am scheduled for early January. My children and their spouses are staying with us for the holidays. My husband and I decide not to tell them until right before they return to their homes (Ohio and California). They are visibly shaken and this was really the hardest part of the ordeal."

And Sharon summarized a major theme in this book when she evaluated her feelings to this conclusion: "My biggest fears after my diagnosis were deformity, chemo, and loss of lymph nodes. I feel fortunate that it was actually relatively easy except for the emotional distress. Physically it was easier than emotionally."

Most of the women found some emotional relief in turning their attention to treatment options. Elaine stated:

"The words you don't want to hear from your doctor are, 'You have cancer.' Immediately you think the worst. You say to yourself, 'No, not me; there must be some mistake.' You go for a second opinion and once again are told you do have cancer. Next, you discuss treatments and options with your doctor. I was told that I have breast cancer and surgery would be the best choice."

Judith, whom you met in Chapter 2, described her painful experience this way:

"I called my surgeon in Kalamazoo. He had done my previous breast needle aspirations but I couldn't get an appointment to see him for 4 weeks, which was in early September. He did an aspiration at that time and no liquid was found. He then did a core needle biopsy, which brought me off the table as he hadn't deadened it enough and it was extremely painful. I had not previously had anything hurt that much and he couldn't understand my reaction. He was pretty sure it was cancerous and gave me a booklet about breast cancer and said he would get back to me when the pathology reports came back. That took another week. He finally called me on Wednesday afternoon and told me the tissue was cancerous and that there was another spot on the right breast that was suspicious and that the radiologist would get in touch with me for further tests. I waited until Friday noon and hadn't heard from them. They say it is important to catch cancer early, so it was frustrating to wait 5–6 weeks to be diagnosed. Because of the puckering that was present I was sure it was cancer but it still was a shock when the doctor called me and told me it was. I sat down on the end of our bed and cried and said, "Why me? It's not fair."

The diagnosis of breast cancer sometimes comes as a surprise. Imagine how Eve felt:

"It was the end of October 1999 and I had a ticket in my pocket to visit my only daughter in the United States. At that time I was a happy grandmother on pension after 27 years of work in Israel. I got an unexpected invitation to get a mammogram. I didn't think about it, but it was time to do it. I went just to have it done without thinking that something can be wrong. After the mammogram they told me to wait and then I had to do it again. They found a small lump in my right breast. At the same time I had a needle biopsy and it was cancer.

The doctor told me that I have a small lump in my right breast and I need a lumpectomy. I told my oncologist that my close family is living in the United States and I will get my treatment there. I needed my daughter's support. I sent a fax to my family that I needed an appointment with a surgeon/oncologist in Detroit as soon as possible. I arrived in Detroit with my mammogram and two direct smears from Tel Aviv. However Dr. V., my surgeon, did a needle biopsy and it was not malignant. He told me that he had to do a lump biopsy to find out what is going on."

In some of the questionnaire responses, like Eve's above, the fear was understated, but as with Sharon's response below we can still appreciate the emotion:

"On the fourth of July 2001, after 11 years of hormone replacement therapy for menopause symptoms, I detected a lump in my left breast. For some reason I didn't suspect it to be cancer. My doctor agreed, but nevertheless sent me for a mammogram. The radiologist concurred that it was a benign area, but saw that two dots of calcification had appeared since my last screening in December. She thought it would prove to be simply changes in cells with age (62), but it needed to be investigated. I was sent to HFH Main Campus for a needle biopsy but was turned away after all my anxiety and schedule juggling because my breasts are too small for that procedure. A surgical biopsy was performed shortly afterwards. The results were positive for the area of calcification and negative for the lump, which also was removed. I was referred to the breast clinic at HFH."

She mentioned her anxiety once, but we can see the shift from her reluctance to believe to an anxious waiting that all cancer patients can identify with.

The women who responded to the questionnaire, however, were able to move beyond their fears, thanks in part to the knowledgeable, caring, nurturing, and understanding way they were dealt with by their doctors and nurses. They moved from fear of the unknown to the beginning of understanding, and they could begin to actively participate in the process of treatment and recovery. Sally Cole-Saul emphasized, "How much better I felt once I felt informed and had made my decisions. Even before the second surgery, I began to feel better once I had evaluated options and made a decision on the procedures I would have done."

The importance of health care professionals in the emotional responses of breast cancer victims is emphasized again and again. Hardeep wrote, "After the lumpectomy, Dr. Nathanson was very upbeat and had great news—'Margins are clear' and 'lymph nodes are clean.' These were very uplifting words." She concluded, "The doctors are very reassuring."

And Rita noted:

"I cannot say I was shocked. My mother, father, and brother had been diagnosed with cancer. I was dismayed. Dr. Nathanson was calm and a little surprised. I knew I was at the right place to face my illness. Thank you so much, Dr. Nathanson, Wanda, and the Breast Care Center."

The realization that she was at "the right place" was directly attributed to the people she met, though she does not specify what these people did.

Isamay gained a similar confidence from the professionals she met:

"Well, to say I was shocked would be an understatement. After all, I am one of those once-a-year mammogram gals! How did I feel? Angry, upset, surprised, sorry for myself. After some calming conversation and realistic advice, I knew the course I would take. Later that same day, I kept my appointment with the surgeon. Because I was over the shock of the news, we were able to determine what procedure was going to be best for me. So my internist and surgeon reinforced confidence and a positive frame of mind."

It's important that the conversation was both "calming" and "realistic." The positive frame of mind that is so helpful to recovery can't be built on a house of cards, and the confidence has to be based on a realistic understanding of what is going to happen. As Isamay put it, "My greatest fear was the unknown. Once I was diagnosed and understood what was happening, I think I developed a very positive attitude." And Gwen said, "Dr. Nathanson explained my treatment in an understandable language."

The empathy of health care professionals is important. Beverly reported, "Dr. M. was a very kind, understanding man. He said to me, 'I do not have cancer but I can empathize with what you must be going through.'" But empathy alone is not sufficient. We see the same mix of reassurance and realism in the experience of Yvonne:

"Like most women who have been diagnosed with breast cancer, my first reactions on being told I had a malignant tumor were surprise, fear, and 'Oh my God, what am I going to do?' and 'How will I cope with this?' Looking back, I found the first few weeks probably the most difficult of the whole experience. It took me a few days to digest the news before I could go forward, then decided the only thing to do was to meet this challenge head on. What doctors to choose, what form of treatment to choose, etc. were just a few of the many questions to be faced. I was fortunate to have had the same primary care physician whom I trusted for many years and I consulted with him with regard to the best doctors for my situation. Once I felt I was in the care of the best doctors, things seemed to get a little easier.

"The best advice I got in the early stages was from one of Dr. Nathanson's nurses who came back into the examination room after my consultation with the doctor who had to give me that bad news, gave me a hug, and said to me, 'The best advice I can give you is 'to make up your mind that the next year will be a shitty [her words, not mine] one, you will feel bad, lose your hair, spend a lot of time in doctors' offices, feel like your life is out of control, etc., etc., etc., but do everything the doctors tell you and know at the end of that year you can put it all behind you and get on with your life.' I can't tell you how many times during that next year I remembered those words—they truly were a big help to me. '*It will be over in a year.*' And you know what, she was right."

Her trusted primary care physician—not an oncologist or breast cancer surgeon—gave her an important voice of reassurance. She was not on her own. And the nurse, in her own way, gave her a very different but even more important kind of reassurance.

Note the same mix of personal comfort and realism in Beverly's account:

"When my husband and I met the doctor, who is so kind, easy to talk to, and has a very soothing voice, he told us the results of the biopsy and talked to us about the sentinel lymph node biopsy with a lumpectomy and 6 year study follow-up. He brought in two oncologists to speak to and explain the procedure involved."

The realism here is not as graphic as "your next year will be a shitty one," but it is based on the fact that experts will be involved who will provide more than a soothing tone of voice. The result was very much like what the Margaret described: "Due to the doctors, nurses, and therapists, I was *scared* but knew *we* could handle it. The doctor helped me get over my initial shock. He explained fully all the ramifications—what may *or* may not happen." The significance of the "we" in Margaret's account is reinforced in Heidi's story below:

"Having experienced invasive breast cancer in 1990, followed by a mastectomy of my right breast and having been informed that a ductal carcinoma in situ means a noninvasive cancer, I accepted this condition, remained calm and positive, and was confident that my medical team would find the best solution to treat me.

"I cannot really say that I felt shocked. Every year, after my first experience with breast cancer, I was grateful that my annual mammogram did not show any sign of recurrence, but I knew that there was a possibility for another cancer.

"My meetings with doctors and nurses at the Breast Clinic were most informative, helpful, and most of all, very assuring and personal. My husband accompanied me, and we were able to ask questions, state our concerns, and come to a decision of treatment that I felt was best and comfortable for me (with doctor's agreement). We felt satisfied that we discussed everything we wanted to know."

Note that she spoke about "my medical team" and how important it was for her, together with her husband, to discuss and understand "everything we wanted to know."

In many cases, the feeling of reassurance that the patient achieved was caused by a combination of the doctor's tone of voice and the patient's own understanding of what was happening and was going to happen. Sally W. had a difficult struggle at first, but note how her tone changed when she began to describe the sentinel node biopsy:

"Dr. Nathanson was a nice looking man. His accent sounds like Australian but he was from South Africa. His first question to me was, 'You found this?' I said yes. He said, 'Nice catch.' He proceeded to explain the biopsy. I would be awake and he would numb a small area near the tumor site. He would make a small cut and this probe would clip pieces of the tumor to determine if it was benign or cancerous. He showed me the instrument. I was numbed and the first of several biopsies were taken. The noise is something they should warn you about if they don't want you to jump. It can really give you a start. If you have ever had your ears pierced you know the 'clang' noise I'm talking about. When it was over I asked when I could get the results. This was Thursday and the results can usually be gotten in a couple of days. Naturally, the weekend got in the way of that. He said I could call next week on Wednesday or Thursday. It was all too much. I couldn't talk. I just hung my head and cried. I must have made him feel bad. Before he left he told me he would try to retrieve the results by Friday night. He also told me he doesn't like to make phone calls on this matter, but he would if I insisted.

"I was in a zombie state most of Friday. About 3 P.M. I was on pins and needles. Really I expected he wouldn't call because it was getting late. At 9:30 P.M. when the phone rang I almost jumped out of my skin because the phone was on my lap as we watched TV. It was Dr. Nathanson. I could hear in his tone of voice right away that it was not good news. 'My dear,' he said, 'it is cancer.' As he was telling me about the size and the path we would take my hearing started to have a funny low ringing. Was I going to faint? Listen to him stupid. I heard the voice of logic at last. It's about 1 cm. This indicated surgery and probably radiation and possible chemotherapy. Make an appointment with my secretary as soon as possible and I will explain a new procedure I would like to do. This procedure called Sentinel Node Biopsy has not yet been approved for standard treatment. It would require a signed release to have it done.

"At my appointment, a lady who already had surgery came in to talk to me and gave me a kit for post-op. The kit contained a rope, hmm (for hanging myself?), a rubber ball, and lots of reading material and business cards. Dr. Nathanson came into explain his new technique, which was featured on Minds of Medicine the very next year on TV.

"He started with a drawing, which really simplified things. 'After we create your incision we inject blue dye around the tumor. We then trace the flow of the dye to the first lymph node that turns blue. We remove that node and have it tested. If it comes back positive (cancer) we remove all the other armpit lymph nodes. If the first node is clear we remove no more lymph nodes and we are done. The old way you lost most of your lymph nodes under your arm, which helped increase your recuperation time and complications. We have to wait for a clean margin on the tumor. If it isn't clean at the margin we have to go in and take more out, until we get a clean margin.' It sounded like a brilliant plan to me and we set a date for surgery.

"I was lucky the first lymph node was clear. There was no spread."

Linda N.'s experience was similar:

"After reviewing my mammogram, Dr. Nathanson suggested that I would be a candidate for a sentinel lymph node biopsy, a procedure that I was familiar with through written articles, but now would experience first hand. If a patient can be a candidate for this procedure, it can be a very wonderful experience. If the sentinel node is cancer free, removing any additional nodes is unnecessary. Recovery from the surgery is much easier and faster with no long-term complications. I thank Dr. N. and his confidence in this procedure every day. Isn't it amazing that a diagnosis as terrifying as cancer can involve a surgery with an almost instantaneous recovery time!"

In both Sally W.'s and Linda N.'s cases, the understanding of the procedure provided a sense of reassurance. Nothing is as frightening as the unknown.

Sally Cole-Saul showed a similar emotional turn:

"When I was first diagnosed in 1993, I initially did not believe it, did not want to believe it, because I had been so focused on health and exercise. I went through a bit of screaming and kicking at the time. Once I acknowledged that I did have cancer, I just wanted to get rid of it and be done with it ASAP. When diagnosed again in 1998, I felt distraught, angry and that it was just plain not fair. Subsequently, my husband and I changed our focus to research for the best approach. This was a very stressful and emotional challenge at the time because we were both working full time in responsible positions, and my cancer became the number one priority in our lives."

The shift to research was a constructive path that many women followed.

Note how Jennie also moved from shock to confidence, thanks in large part to a reassuring human voice:

"I went for my yearly mammogram and the results were to have an incision biopsy. Once the biopsy was taken, I then saw Dr. G. He came into the room and said, 'I have good and bad news. Good news is the left breast is OK, but the right breast has the lump, which should be removed.' I would need radiation for 6 weeks.

"Just the month before I lost my brother with lung cancer, who had chemo and radiation! I said, 'If I have the mastectomy would I need any treatments?' The doctor said no.

"It was a shock to hear the word 'cancer.' Inside me, I felt the world had just fallen through. My husband was in the room with me and the nurse W. talked with us. She gave us a lot of confidence. After a few minutes, I made myself understand that I wasn't the first person to have cancer!"

Nobody wants to discover the truth about her breast cancer, but sometimes the reality simply fights its way through. Listen to Susan's story of discovery and the way she made a constructive emotional transition:

"I noticed a small lump, the size of a pea, which looked and felt like a bruise, near the surface of my breast. Thinking it was a bruise and would dissipate into the tissue, I waited for 3 weeks. But when it didn't go away, I went to see a doctor. At this stage, it was the size of a marble. The doctor took a needle biopsy and said he would do a mammogram and ultrasound when he saw me for my annual checkup, which was in 2 months time. The needle aspiration/biopsy came back negative. Two months later, when I returned for my annual checkup, the lump was now the size of a golf ball. The doctor sent me for an emergency mammogram and ultrasound the same day and 3 days later I was referred to a surgeon as the radiologist 'didn't like what he saw.'

"At this stage, I still wasn't concerned because there was no history of cancer on either of my parents' sides of the family. Although I know that not having a history of cancer in your family doesn't mean anything, I still felt less 'vulnerable.'

"When I saw the surgeon, she had already seen the mammogram and ultrasound reports. She took one look at me and said, 'You have cancer.' I have read about the shock of being told you have cancer, but nothing can prepare you for this moment. My first thoughts were, 'Are you talking to me? Is there someone else in the room with us—behind me perhaps?'

"She [the doctor] was extremely gentle and compassionate. She gave me the facts in a straightforward manner. I asked if I could make notes because I was unlikely to remember everything as I was in shock, but she assured me they would be giving everything to me in writing as well. She asked whether I had any questions and said I should call if I thought of anything later. One of the questions I remember asking was whether or not I'd have to have chemotherapy. I was calm leaving her office but when relaying the information to my husband on the phone, that was when I broke down and cried. I was in shock, frightened, but also reassured by the information the doctor had shared with me. I also kept reminding myself that the treatment now is so much better than it was even just 10 years ago. I went straight back to work where everyone—men and women—were supportive and empathetic. One of the women had gone through treatment a year previously and I found it comforting to speak with her."

Susan moves from shock to breaking down to rallying with the aid of the informative support of her doctor and the additional support of friends and coworkers.

Of course, every patient's experience with their physicians is not always so positive. Beatrice, whose discovery of a lump we saw in Chapter 2, described this unfortunate event:

"So after the second set of mammograms, they asked if I would stay for an ultrasound. The radiologist entered while I was still lying down. Without introduction, he became angry with me. He asked me in a cold, clipped manner, 'Didn't you have anyone examine your breast manually this year?' Obviously he had not been trained to give bad news, or he simply chose to blame the victim.

"I found myself trying to calm him by explaining that other pressing physical problems took precedence. Thus, I had missed the 6-month manual checkup. He didn't ask what the other medical concerns were. He is the only crass, boorish doctor I have ever met. This hospital is known for its excellent work on the doctor–patient relationships. I asked others how he could be like this. I was told that he often found an excuse to miss the workshops or seminars. It was known that he needed this information. What a shame that he was the one person giving the results of these tests.

"And of course his gruffness was the first concrete sign that there was a tumor. My feelings of sureness that a malignancy would be present didn't make me worry. Whatever needed to be done would be done. I would have opted for surgery without further tests but more information had to be put together."

Beatrice's experience appears to be the exception rather than the rule. Most doctors are trained to deal in a more appropriate way than the one described here. In fact, there is not always a magically correct way to break the news as Lucille's story illustrates:

"Well, here I am a healthy 65-year-old with no family history of breast cancer. However, in October 1998, after my yearly mammogram, I was advised to see a cancer surgeon. A urologist friend at Henry Ford West Bloomfield said that Dr. Nathanson was the best. After a consultation, I was sent for a stereotactic biopsy. Now the journey begins.

"This was a big new adventure for someone who had not been near a hospital, except for childbirth. A few days later Dr. N. called with the news that it's cancer.

"I wasn't surprised and said, 'What's next?'

"'Can you wait till January after the holidays, for a lumpectomy and possible radiation?'

"So, brave person that I was, I reported in early January at Henry Ford Hospital in downtown Detroit at 7 A.M. for wire localization. Little did I know what came next! Two hours later, after being in compression most of the time, I was left there with three wires sticking up out of my breast. By then I had lost my place in line for the OR. Six hours later, with no food or drink, I was ready to leave, wires and all, but they caught me before I could escape. The surgery was a shock and I hoped that was the end of it.

"My next meeting came after a few days later with Dr. N. and my husband. He walked in and said, 'Good news, no nodes [he had done a sentinel node biopsy], but you must have a mastectomy.' With that comment, my stomach went plop and I fell apart. I had cared for my aunt and saw what she looked like for 25 years after a mastectomy. I said, 'No way, I give up.'

"His comment was, 'You will be as flat as a 5-year-old.' I wasn't laughing."

I am troubled by the 6-hour delay and by the "I wasn't laughing" in response to the doctor's poorly timed attempt at humor.

A few patients, for different reasons, did not feel any fear. From Heidi:

"There is no real fear in my life. What happens, happens. I lived through World War II (as a child), I immigrated to the United States on my own initiative, and so far I have 'conquered' my health problems. Yes, there is concern and I worry from time to time. With having two different kinds of breast cancers and skin cancer, there is the possibility of ovarian cancer. I gave consent to a DNA test that is in process with Dr. Q. and a genetic counselor."

And from Jennie:

"I didn't have any fear. I felt whatever illness came to me would be taken care of through my surgeon and his staff who work together and made me comfortable. In my mind this is what God is giving me. I will do everything to get better. With prayers and faith we take one day at a time."

These stoical responses, however, are the exceptions.

The comfort that some patients take in an understanding of their disease and the process of their treatment was evident in a number of responses to our questionnaire. The following account by Eve is typical:

"On 11/16/99 was my first surgery, the right breast excisional biopsy. The lump was a well-differentiated invasive ductal carcinoma; one margin positive for ductal carcinoma in situ. The tumor was greater than 1 cm but not bigger than 2 cm. Dr. V. told me that now I needed a second surgery to find out if the lymph nodes were clear and to clean the place around the lump biopsy margins in my breast. When the discussions went on about my surgery and my treatment, Dr. Nathanson, the director of the Breast Center, came to see me for a few moments and told me, 'You don't need a mastectomy. You will have the same chances of surviving with the lumpectomy.' His words were music to my ears. It was exactly what I wanted to hear because all my life I felt as a satisfied female and my breast was a part of it. I felt that my treatment will not be easy, but I have to do what I have to do! Thank you Dr. N., you gave me trust in Henry Ford Hospital.

"My second surgery took place on 11/19/1999. Dr. V. told me that he checked twelve lymph nodes and one came out positive. It is not so good but not so bad either. I needed chemotherapy because of the positive lymph node. He talked to Dr. S. and I went to see him. We made an appointment for the next week and I told him that I wanted to bring my daughter (a physician) with me to talk about my treatment. I was excited and the expertise of Dr. S., Senior Staff Physician Hematology/Oncology Division, made me feel better. I realized that there are a lot of women in my situation and there is a good way to treat the breast cancer today. The fact that I arrived to see Dr. S. with my doctor daughter gave me more confidence in the decisions I had to make in my case. Dr. S. was short and firm about my case and he wrote down the path I have to go through my treatment: chemotherapy every 21 days, 8 times (Adriamycin and Cytoxan IV every 21 days, 4 times, then Taxol IV every 21 days, 4 times). Done in 6 months."

Several things strike me here. First, the medical language is obvious, and in fact, many women were conversant about the nature of their cancers and the medications they were taking. Second, the patient is very clear about who is making the medical decisions—and it's not only her doctor! And third, the patient is not especially reassured by her physician's soothing tone of voice, but instead she seems to appreciate his being "short and firm about my case." Her reassurance derives more from having a clear understanding of "the path I have to go through my treatment." Gone are the days when patients were ignorant and passive. As a physician, I am thankful for the change—especially thankful for the shared decision-making responsibility.

It's important to remember that the diagnosis of breast cancer occurs in the context of ongoing lives with family, friends and coworkers. D'Anna, another voice from Chapter 2, told her story this way:

"I was given the diagnosis of breast cancer at 5:00 P.M. on Friday, December 17. I had to wait until Dr. Nathanson was out of surgery. We had dinner planned for that evening with two other families, friends of mine from work. My good friend, David, and his family were already there when I got home, so they heard the diagnosis at the same time my husband did. We ate dinner and drove through the Wayne County Light Fest on Hines Drive as planned. Later that evening, I called my parents to tell them. My mother started crying, and I thought, 'Please don't do this to me. I need you.' The next evening was our Division's Christmas party. I didn't want to be a downer, but I knew I would have to tell everyone. And everyone was waiting for the news.

"The next Thursday (the day before Christmas Eve), my husband and I met my parents for the breast cancer clinic at Henry Ford Hospital where we spent the day talking to various nurses and doctors. They scheduled my surgery for the following Thursday, December 29. Dr. N. told me I was a good candidate for lumpectomy and radiation, and he wanted to do a Sentinel Node Biopsy, where they would inject a radioactive tracer and a blue dye to find the first lymph node that drains the breast area. If there was no cancer in that node, then I would be spared the removal of other nodes and the problems that could cause in the future. I had known the scientists in his lab and had lunched with them for years, so I knew a little bit about what they were working on. I thought it was so cool that something they had actually researched in the lab had matured into a procedure done on patients in the OR!

"After the clinic, my husband and I went straight back to our church for a dress rehearsal. He is the Director of Music and I was in a play we were doing on Christmas Eve. The play was called 'Twinkle,' and it was about the star that God chose to be over the manger. The pastor had given me a couple of lines to sing, 'It just takes a little faith and you can move a mountain, Believe and you can light up the sky.' "

I'm impressed with the way D'Anna, like many who accomplished the ordinary miracle of cancer recovery, was able to draw upon her life-context for strength and reassurance.

Sometimes the health care institution can itself play an important role in creating or supporting a positive attitude in those just diagnosed with breast cancer. Isamay gave a clear description of the approach we use at Henry Ford Hospital—and her enthusiasm for our approach:

"Five years ago next month, I had my annual mammogram at the Fairlane Clinic. Within a few days, I received a phone call indicating that a follow-up visit was necessary because an abnormality appeared. I phoned immediately and secured the referrals from my primary physician (Dr. D.F., Fairlane Clinic) for the Multi-Disciplinary Breast Clinic for evaluation and treatment. This tumor board, as I remember it being called, was the greatest! Husband Bob and I and six other patients arrived at the Main Campus early one appointed morning. A brief explanation of the process was given, and each patient (and her accompanying friend) was assigned an examination room. Then, one by one, a representative of each discipline involved in the treatment came to see me. It was like 'one stop shopping' because it eliminated the need for multiple appointments in various departments of the hospital. This is a fabulous concept! The entire process was rapid and efficient. In a week and a half, I had my appointment with the surgeon (Dr. F., Main Campus); he recommended a needle biopsy or a stereotactic core biopsy. I really wanted the test that very moment—but took the first available appointment, which was for the stereo-tactic core biopsy. This occurred the next week. A week after the procedure, I had an appointment with my internist (Dr. F.) early in the morning. After the 'how are you doings,' I reviewed what had gone on over the prior few weeks. He checked the computer for my test results—returned to the exam room and said, 'It's positive.'"

Keep in mind that her "the greatest" and "fabulous" were written in the context of the diagnosis of breast cancer! Julia called the program "super" because "everyone who participated was helpful."

We see Sonya's experience with the same breast clinic format:

"I am so thankful to be a breast cancer survivor and to tell my story. My story begins with my annual mammogram November 1999. By the end of November, I received a call from my primary care doctor to have a repeat mammogram of my left breast. I decided to wait until after the Christmas holiday to have it done. The repeat x-ray was abnormal. I was told that I should have a biopsy done. After the biopsy, I was given an appointment to the Breast Clinic to get the results of the biopsy. The nurse gave all of the women in the conference room a bag with books and other information about breast cancer and different treatments. The first doctor I talked with was the surgeon, Dr. T. He told me he was sorry to tell me that the tumor was cancer. For a brief moment I just felt numb. No, I didn't cry. Just felt numb. Dr. T. helped me overcome the initial shock by explaining to me that when breast cancer is found and treated early, the chances for survival are better. Those words of encouragement made me feel better. The last doctor I talked with was Dr. Nathanson. I had chosen to have a lumpectomy."

We don't see the explicit kudos here for the clinic, but we do see how it worked well for this patient.

Hardeep had a similar experience:

"I did not go back to my internist [who first diagnosed breast cancer]. I went directly to the oncologists, radiologists, and two surgeons. They were very supportive, reassuring me that I had options, that my prognosis was good, and that many women live on after cancer."

The last sentence shows how a successful transition can be achieved.

Here is Alyce's overview of how the clinic worked for a recently diagnosed patient:

"When I went to the surgeon's office he performed a biopsy and without blinking said I had breast cancer. But he informed me of the Henry Ford Breast Clinic that was held the following day. Approximately seven or eight MDs would observe and consult on my condition. He said I could bring my whole family. I was petrified and shocked. I could not talk. Of course, there was no sleep that night. The next morning at 7 A.M. my daughter, my husband, and I drove to the clinic. When we arrived my son-in-law and granddaughter met us.

"There were six or seven people in attendance at the clinic and an R.N. opened by telling us we would feel better when the day ended. We were each put in a single room with our family and I was shaking badly. As each doctor approached it was somewhat comforting. Each doctor confirmed I would only need a lumpectomy and each one emphasized the ease of the surgery. By the end of the day I was actually smiling, as each member of my family was, and I had total faith knowing I was in good hands. We all left by 4 o'clock feeling very relieved."

The movement from "petrified and shocked" to "actually smiling" was not caused by the fact of the relatively good news that she would "only need a lumpectomy." It's the comforting presence of the team in whose care she was being placed.

Judith attended our clinic after a trip across the state of Michigan. Again we see the experience of breast cancer in the larger context of the patient's life:

"After I heard the news from my doctor on Wednesday, I waited until Friday noon and hadn't heard anything from the radiologist. We had been to Henry Ford Hospital in Detroit numerous times with follow-ups for my husband after his heart transplant. I would pick up information on cancer treatments and what HFHS was doing in the field. I was interested as he is very susceptible to cancer because of his suppressed immune system.

"Early Friday afternoon I found the information I had collected, which included the Breast Clinic, and called the 800 number and spoke to a telephone operator. She asked if I could get my path slides and report, ultrasound and mammogram and doctor reports by the afternoon. I said I would try. I called the three different places and arranged to pick up everything. I called back about 3:30 that afternoon and she asked me to fax my path report to her. She already had an appointment with Dr. L. on Tuesday at 4:30 P.M. The surgeon here in Kalamazoo was concerned that I wanted my records and was going to another facility but he released them.

"We took all my test information and drove to Detroit, which was a $2^1/_2$-hour drive, on Tuesday and met with Dr. L., who I later discovered was the chief surgeon at HFHS. After the examination he said there were two alternatives. He could do another biopsy, which would tell them the same results and have the lumpectomy the following Thursday or we could do the operation this Thursday. We decided to have the surgery that Thursday.

"While there, I went through the breast cancer clinic. As I had already had my surgery, they took me to a clinic room and I spoke with the radiation and oncology specialists. I didn't see the surgeon as that part was over. The group had already met after my surgery and reviewed my case and they had the recommendations all mapped out, which were 6 months of chemo and 33 radiation treatments. I did see the social worker but had no need for any of the services. The telephone operator stopped by while I was there to meet me and say 'hi.' She is a super person to have in that position.

"The program was very informative and if time had allowed it would have been better to have gone through that first before surgery but it all worked out fine."

Note how important to Judith was the personal touch from the telephone operator, who at first was just a voice from an 800 number.

For some, such as Lizabeth, the shift to a positive attitude takes the form of a wry sense of humor:

"I was diagnosed with breast cancer on the Friday before Labor Day in 1999. I was planning to leave the next day for a 2-week vacation in Greece or Turkey. After some discussion with Dr. E., it looked like my vacation was not going to happen. But after some more consideration, Dr. E. agreed to help me meet with all the doctors and get all of the tests that I needed. I spent the day walking around the clinic meeting with people and getting information (more, probably, than I could digest). I left for vacation the next day. After spending the day in New York, we arrived at the Intercontinental Hotel in Athens. As we were cleaning up and unpacking, the room began to shake, escalating to pretty violent movement. A serious earthquake had struck Athens and we were 6 miles from the epicenter. Surviving that, we traveled through Greece and went to Turkey—where we experienced another earthquake. In 1 week I was diagnosed with cancer and experienced two earthquakes—seemed like the biblical plagues and earthquakes. At that point I assumed I would live—there had been too many easy chances to get me."

Many of the women made an important transition when they moved past their initial shock to a more constructive response, using whatever internal and external resources they could draw upon. In doing so, they came to see the diagnosis as the first step toward recovery.

4

CASE STUDY—SALLY SAWYER: "A LIFE BEYOND CANCER"

Sally Sawyer is a woman in her late 60s who has the gift of a powerful sense of her life despite the temporary interruption she experienced from her breast cancer treatment. Deeply involved in the theater, she nurtured this important part of her identity by continuing to act and write during her treatment. People with breast cancer are no longer passively compliant, blindly doing what they are told, when they are told. Sally's determination to further her personal artistic life, despite the time constraints imposed by her breast cancer treatments, made her feel as if there was meaning in her existence. She is fun and funny and is one of those people who manage to counteract problems and difficulties with humor.

She presented the account of her experience with breast cancer dramatically, through dialogue, as befits a survivor so committed to the theater.

JANUARY 2001

"Please Lord, *please!*"

I squeezed my eyelids tightly facing the long row of icy beige lockers at West Bloomfield's Henry Ford Hospital mammogram center.

"If it be thy will, let this cup pass from me. Please!"

I realized I was talking out loud when one lady sitting outside the changing area cleared her throat uncomfortably. Another whispered audibly to her, "I wonder if she got bad news."

"Janet," the technician who took my x-ray had said, "the radiologist wants to see you before you leave." At first I did not respond. "Janet" is the name on my Certificate of Registration. I'm called "Sally." I'm adopted. I have many first names.

Turning around, I replied, "Do you mean Mrs. S.?"

"Yes, Janet." She didn't catch my innuendo. I don't feel on a first name basis with someone half my age that really doesn't know who I am or what I'm called.

Her mouth smiled, so I followed her to a dark booth where the radiologist had my mammogram on the viewing screen. He called me "Mrs. S." and shook my hand.

"Sit down. I have something to show you." Fear crept over me and the room suddenly felt cold.

"Do you see this dark spot in your left breast?" He pointed with his pen.
"Yes."

"That is a suspicious area. I'd like you to have a new type of biopsy." Being an R.N. didn't help me to read the x-ray. It all looked lumpy and bumpy to me . . . except for the dark spot. "Check the front desk and they'll schedule you."

I thanked him and thought, "What an awful job he has . . . telling women they may have cancer!"

The lady at the front desk told me the earliest I could have this new biopsy in our area would be in 2 weeks.

"What will my family think?" I wondered on the way home.

"Wait 2 weeks? That's ridiculous," remarked my husband, Jerry, an M.D. He obtained the x-rays and hand delivered them to Mt. Clemens General Hospital. The following day I was at Mt. Clemens at 8 A.M., lying flat on my stomach. My left breast hung through a hole in the examination table.

"Didn't know I had enough to hang," I said to the nurse. She smiled and told me I had "q.s." (quantity sufficient).

Soon a doctor came in and numbed my breast and proceeded to make a series of about twenty to thirty jabs into the breast to extract areas for biopsy. Fortunately for me, I neither saw nor felt a thing.

After I was off the table, I peeked into a small dish, seeing something that looked like red spaghetti. A person from the lab labeled and whisked the specimen away. The doctor reappeared, in a suit.

"We may have taken all the cancer tissue in the area," he said. "It looks good so far." This was the first time a medical person said "cancer" to me.

My appointment with Dr. N. was 1 week hence. Two days a week I worked at Barnes & Noble as "Story Lady" in the children's area and three evenings a week I was rehearsing for the Cole Porter musical, *Anything Goes.*

"How can you stand waiting for the biopsy report?" friends asked.

"Frankly, I don't have much time to think about it, with play rehearsals and preparing for Story Time."

My husband, Jerry, accompanied me to see Dr. N. The nurse put a box of Kleenex on the table where I sat. "Hmm," I wondered. "Is that a bad omen?"

Dr. N. came in, looked at the article I was reading in *The Atlantic Monthly* and was introduced to my husband. Then he looked at the biopsy report and asked, " How do you feel today?"

"Actually, quite well and very lucky. I've had about ten breast biopsies over the years, and so far they've all been negative."

"Well, you're not so lucky this time. The biopsy came back positive."

The nurse handed me a Kleenex. My husband looked concerned.

"I still feel lucky, Dr. N. My birth mother died at 31, of stomach cancer. I'm more than twice that age now."

"What are the options?" asked Jerry.

Dr. N. looked at me. "You can have a total mastectomy with no radiation . . . or a lumpectomy with radiation. You may also need chemo. However, I'm doing a study using a relatively new method called 'sentinel node biopsy' in combination with a lumpectomy. We check and see if the cancer has spread to the lymph nodes. With this method you must have radiation . . . and possibly, chemotherapy, depending on how large the cancer area is. If you like, you can be in this study."

I paused a moment to absorb the shock that cancer was dwelling in my body. I was stunned but did not cry.

"Let me think about this before I decide."

"The method is up to you," Dr. N. said. "I want it to be *your* decision."

"Why don't you have the mastectomy?" my husband suggested. "Then you won't have to keep worrying about each new lump."

"If your wife were having this operation, what would you suggest to her?" I asked Dr. N.

"I would suggest the lumpectomy . . . with the sentinel node biopsy."

"If I have the sentinel node biopsy and a lumpectomy, will I still have a nipple?"

"Yes."

"You know, I've always wanted to be in a study, but I was never accepted because I have no family history."

"You can be in *my* study."

"How soon can I have the operation?"

"When do you want it?"

"Yesterday will be fine."

Dr. N. smiled. "I don't think we can do it that quickly. I'll check the schedule at Henry Ford downtown. That's where I do my surgery. We'll try to arrange it for next week." He shook hands with us and said, "See you soon."

On returning home we told our son. Dan said, "Do anything it takes to recover, mom."

I called our daughter, Theresa, on Long Island. She was shocked and said, "I guess I'd better get checked, too!"

"That's a good idea, but I don't think you are as likely a candidate as I am. You started your periods at 14 and have been able to breast feed all your babies."

"But I was 33 when I had my first baby. Let me talk to Dad."

So went the first day, knowing I had cancer.

The following evening was play rehearsal. Afterward I told the director, "You'd better cast someone else in my part. I have breast cancer and will have it operated on soon."

"How soon?" she said looking concerned.

"Probably next week."

"Well, this is only January. The play isn't till March. We'll wait for you."

Pleasantly surprised, I said, "Then, I'll see that I'm well enough to do it. I love that role. I've never been a comedic antagonist before."

"*Wing & a Prayer Players* will help you. Don't quit. You're hilarious in the part."

A few days later, my husband and I attended a multiple doctor conference to discuss my *early* breast cancer. We were happy to hear they considered it *early.* Having them all together was a blessing both in time and knowing they were working together.

At Barnes & Noble I told my manager and fellow workers about my operation. My immediate supervisor's eyes teared.

"My mother died of breast cancer last year."

"I'm sorry to hear that," I told her. "I feel fine and look at the surgery as just a detour that must be followed for now." Then I went back to meet Devin Skillion (Channel 4 anchor man) and gather the Story Hour children to hear him read his newest book, *Fibblestax.*

Wednesday, January 31, 2001, I had the lumpectomy and sentinel node biopsy. Afterward, semi-awake, I heard Dr. N. talking with my husband.

"It all looks very clear and we didn't have to put in a drain." Dr. N. apologized for having taken so much tissue.

"That's all right. I didn't have much to begin with. A little less won't matter."

"Do you have any pain?"

"No. When can I go home?"

"Soon."

That evening, I slept on the family room couch by the fireplace. Our cat, Muffy, slept on my stomach. I could doze off and still be within a few steps of the bathroom. My throat was very sore, but still no breast pain. Now, if only I could urinate! Early the next morning a doctor from Ford called about my condition.

"I'm fine and have no pain."

"Good, I'm glad to hear that."

"But my throat is very sore and I can't urinate."

"Your sore throat is from the tube they put down. Now, I want you to drink lots of fluids. Be constantly sipping on something. If you don't pass some water in 12 hours, come in and we'll catheterize you."

"No way!" I thought, and began the "force fluids" regime.

By 6:00 that evening, feeling 12 months pregnant, I turned on two faucets, sat upon the throne, and thought liquid thoughts . . . like, Niagara Falls! I pushed on my bladder. Within a few minutes, I relaxed and finally felt a few drops.

"Praise God from whom all blessings flow," I croaked, trying to sing.

The following week Dr. N. looked at my dressing and told me my lymph nodes were negative. I was started on Tamoxifen and put back on all the medications I had taken before surgery. Soon I was to start radiation.

That afternoon, washing dishes, an ice-loaded gutter fell on top of my garden window over the sink. Incredibly, it shattered the "inside" layer of glass leaving the "outside" unscathed! Shards of glass were all over my arms, the sink, and floor. Unprepared for the loud noise, I started crying uncontrollably.

"Boy, are you stupid," I thought. "You cry at a broken window and make jokes about your cancer."

By the middle of February, I was back to everything I had done before the surgery. However, I was tired and needed frequent naps. Unfortunately, I had taken myself off thyroid, thinking it was part of the medications to be discontinued before surgery. I went back to work 2 days a week at Barnes & Noble and continued singing with the Birmingham Musicale. I attended play rehearsal, frequent doctor's appointments, and managed to cast and present a reading for Michigan Playwrights.

Knowing I would be even more fatigued once radiation began, I pleaded with the radiotherapy attendants to have it started as soon as possible. I was especially concerned that the last treatments would coincide with play performance dates in March.

"There are patients just as sick as you are, Janet. I can't bump them out of their scheduled treatments just for you."

"Well, how about starting me the week *after* my play is over."

"No, no!... You must start on March 14 and continue daily for 33 treatments... No weekends, of course. This is your life and you are toying with the prospects."

My husband had picked up the phone, hearing the controversy about scheduling. "This is Dr. S. My wife had her surgery in January and she isn't having radiation till the middle of March? Seems to me that after waiting this long, 2 extra weeks wouldn't do any harm."

"No. She must start Wednesday, March 14!"

Grabbing the phone, I hoped to prevent an ugly confrontation. "I must be in for my first treatment on the 14th, but after that... I don't know."

"You *must* continue the treatments as prescribed!"

"Please try to understand. After the play is over on March 24, I'll be a good little girl and do exactly as you say."

Dial tone.

On March 14 I had my first radiation treatment amidst snide and sarcastic remarks from the staff. I said nothing. A nurse who did all the procedural explaining looked at me as I left the treatment area and asked to speak to me.

"Your face is red. Let me take your blood pressure." It registered around 170/90.

"What's bothering you?" she asked.

I told her I had a lead in my church play... a part I've always wanted. The whole cast was depending on me. "I must rest tomorrow... all day. It's opening night."

"Go ahead," she smiled. "And good luck."

When I arrived for treatment the following Monday, I was shuffled off to see a social worker. Apparently I was considered a "difficult" person. She was friendly and seemed to understand my interest in theatre. Her daughter was in a school play at the time.

"I thought you were a playwright."

"Yes, I am. I have my MFA in theatre and write and direct. I enjoy acting sometimes, too . . ."

"Is anything bothering you?"

"Not really, except many things I've wanted all my life are finally coming my way. My cancer is badly timed . . . an interference with my life."

"Do you resent that?"

"Of course, but I'm not going to let cancer take over my life. It's just a 'necessary detour' . . . (There I go . . . using that phrase again!) What I mean is, I have a life beyond cancer. I expect to fulfill all my artistic opportunities . . . just postpone them a bit . . . if possible."

"I understand," she replied. I wish more of the *staff* understood!

"Bring one of your plays with you next time. I'd like to see it."

"Really? I'll bring it and leave it in your office soon. Then, I'm not going to be in consistently till Monday, March the 26th . . . when the play is over."

During the interim, I noticed my right hand began to tremble. I couldn't control it unless I grabbed something very tightly . . . like a teacup.

"You sound like the 'Bells of Saint Mary's,'" Dan quipped, recalling a friend with the same affliction, who rattled toward us with cups of hot tea.

On March 20, my third radiation treatment was over without any of the personnel saying more than necessary. I attempted to get off the treatment table and gasped at the sharp pain in my back. Heads turned my way.

"Please help me get off the table," I requested, arms up. One of the attendants came over offering me her hand.

"That won't do it," I said. "I will still be using my back muscles."

She called her coworker because she herself had a "bad back." The coworker came and I put my arms around her neck.

"If you can get me halfway up," I said, "I'll swing my feet around. Then I can get down by myself."

Surprisingly, she complied. As I was leaving, the first attendant reminded me to tie up my gown in back for the short walk to the dressing room.

"Oh, it's all right. There's no one out there. Besides, being in theatre, I'm used to streaking."

Damn! I bit my tongue. These folks aren't used to my sense of humor. I'll probably have to see the psychologist again for my "indecent exposure tendencies."

By early April, and my thirteenth radiation treatment, I was on better terms with the radiation personnel. I told them I would have to miss the next treatment because a good friend of ours had died in a barn fire in Belmont, Ontario. We were going to the funeral.

"I know exactly where you're talking about," said one of the attendants. "I'm from that part of Canada. Belmont is about 2 miles away."

"I'm concerned about his family. The oldest boy is only 13."

"Don't worry. The farmers help each other . . . for years, sometimes."

"Thank you for your concern," I responded; grateful that someone realized I had a life aside from cancer concerns.

On my return from Canada, I brought a Belmont newspaper for the Canadian attendant. It described our friend's merits and how well he was known and liked . . . how kind he was. He had died in the barn's birthing area trying to save a mother cow and her calf. After this, the tension level in the radiology department dropped to zero. We even became quite friendly.

Later that April, fatigue hit me full blast. Determined not to let it interfere with my life, I continued to work, grabbing naps when and where I could. I even went to Chicago with one of my adult students to see her play premiere in a fell equity house. I slept all the way there and back in the rear seat of her car.

In May I accepted a Creative Writers' in Schools National Endowment grant and taught at Pasteur Elementary in Detroit. I told the teacher who requested me I would be able to work only mornings due to radiation treatments in the afternoon. Maybe she'd better get someone else.

"Don't let that concern you," she said. "My mother is principal of Pasteur and she had a double mastectomy for cancer last year."

As I hung up, I thought happily, "It's so nice to know that people aren't afraid to mention 'cancer' anymore."

One of the high points of my recovery was when Dr. N. chose me to be a subject in 2001 *Minds of Medicine*, a Henry Ford Health System minimagazine. Many people called to offer their sympathy after seeing my picture with my husband in the magazine. I soon had them laughing at this very healthy, near 70-year-old, being a centerfold!"

It is now January 2004, 3 years since my lumpectomy and sentinel node biopsy. I've had the chance to reevaluate my mortality . . . how I fit into the lives of my children and grandchildren, my church, and community activities. I've chiseled down some of the extras and am concentrating on what I *really* want to do with the rest of my life.

As to advice to future cancer patients, I'm not much for giving advice unless asked, but I can tell you what I do. I exercise daily as I have done all my life, eat lots of fruits and vegetables, try to rid life of as much stress as possible, and have routine mammograms and yearly physicals.

Have faith in God, believe that prayer does work; laugh often and love much. Don't think of yourself as a cancer "victim" but a cancer "survivor." As you think, so it will be.

5

SURGERY: "THIS WASN'T BAD"

One might think that the surgery itself might be the most intimidating part of the process of discovering, diagnosing, and treating breast cancer. The responses, however, show a very different reality. Once the shock and fear associated with the unknown future gave way to the concrete process of treatment and recovery, the emotional pain subsided. As Gwen put it, "This wasn't bad, but I was scared. My doctor was great. My recuperation was fast." And Margaret said, "Everything was explained in advance; that helped."

Note what was said and what was not said in the following description from Elaine:

"A mammogram I had taken in January of 2001 showed a suspicious condition in a milk duct of the right breast. After agreeing to surgery (a lumpectomy), it was performed at the end of the month and confirmed that cancer was present. Luckily it was only one and a half centimeters which was good news. The doctor then suggested that more surgery was necessary to check the lymph nodes. This operation was scheduled in February, and I was relieved to hear later that the cancer had not invaded that area. As a precautionary measure to future cancer development, it is customary to have six weeks of radiation treatments five days a week. Radiation therapy is a treatment using high energy rays (such as x-rays) to kill or shrink cancer cells."

Elaine hardly mentioned the surgery itself, but rather the reasons for the surgery and radiation and the prospects of recovery. She was well informed about what was happening and why, she agreed to the procedure, and her attitude was positive and constructive.

In another case, Julia did not need to use her advanced training, but we can sense her confidence in being prepared:

"Surgery was performed by Dr. B. and I thought he did a fantastic job. I was fortunate and did not need to use the drainage procedure we had been trained to handle at the cancer day orientation. I was terribly tired for a period after the surgery. Don't know why except I believe body shock and worry caused it." I love the way she is so involved in understanding what is happening to her.

One of the more positive descriptions of the surgery was this by Ethel: "The surgery to remove the lump and one node was a breeze. Discomfort was minimal, almost nil, and I had no apprehensions. I never experienced edema or depression. Again, Dr. N. was very supportive and explained the procedures along the way. My relationship with Dr. N. was an important part of the total experience." Again and again we see that the relationship with the health care team is an important part of the overall experience.

Many women reported on their surgery with a surprising absence of anxiety, probably because of the amount of preparation they were given. Note Susan's tone of voice:

"I was given the choice of a lumpectomy or a mastectomy and discussed with my surgeon, the fact that I would have a mastectomy if it was necessary, otherwise my choice would be a lumpectomy which she agreed with. I had many medical tests before the surgery. Whilst waiting for my surgery date I carried on my normal schedule and found it was best to keep active and keep my mind busy. The surgery went well. Some of my lymph nodes had had to be removed and I was told I would have to have chemotherapy."

Like Susan, Judith retained her equanimity thanks both to the physicians who were part of her team and her own strength of character:

"We then met with nurse W.S., Coordinator for the Breast Clinic. She arranged a hotel for us and scheduled all the necessary tests I needed for surgery for Wednesday, which was the next morning. We stayed at the Hyatt Regency in Dearborn which was a very nice and relaxing place to spend your time when you are facing surgery for the first time in your life. On Wednesday morning we reported in and had the blood test and chest x-ray. Then we went upstairs and they did an ultrasound of the right breast to see what was there. They did an ultrasound and a needle aspiration which didn't produce anything. Then they used an 18-gauge needle and got some fluid out of it. The spot disappeared and any problems were ruled out with that breast.

"After the tests we went back to the hotel and cruised through the gift shop and ate at one of their restaurants and retired about 10 P.M.

"On Thursday, October 4, we arrived at the Nuclear Medicine Lab at 7 A.M. They inserted the blue dye at the site of the tumor and tracked it to the sentinel lymph node. I was then sent to a waiting room to wait for Dr. L.'s assistant to come and get me for surgery which was at 8:30. I was reading a magazine when at 9 A.M. Dr. L. appeared at the door and asked if I was ready. I told him I thought his assistant was coming to get me. He said all of his assistants were busy so he came to get me and the information from the nuclear lab. Not many chief surgeons would have done this. I found him to be a very compassionate person.

"When I got to the pre-op room, things moved quickly as I was a half hour late. Everything went well except the IV, which the fellow couldn't get in my right hand. Another person tried and it went fine. The last thing I remember was the bright lights in the operating room and having a mask put over my face.

"I woke up in the recovery room about 2:30 P.M. and I had a very hard time keeping my eyes open. The first thing I saw was my husband standing there smiling and he handed me a little red-spotted toy dog. This was the first time I had ever been in a hospital other than having my two daughters. I had been through a lot with my husband's surgeries but it was much different being the patient.

"Dr. L. came in and said they had to take a larger amount of the breast as the tumor was 1 cm on the top but 2.5 cm on the bottom. They took two margins to be sure the surrounding tissues were clear. It was the upper limit for a lumpectomy. He also said he removed the sentinel lymph node and some small ones around it. He apologized for what he had to do as he knew I was expecting a small incision and scar. I was a little nauseated after waking up but it went away. They had removed the IV and I still wasn't doing very well. I said to the nurse maybe I should stay another day. He said they would have to put the IV back in and I said never mind I was going home. The IV hurt more than anything. I don't like needles even for drawing blood and in the past had fainted.

"The discharge person came with the wheelchair and I had to go to the bathroom before leaving which was an experience as I didn't have the complete use of my legs and I had a hard time getting from the wheelchair to the stool. But I made it and at 6:00 P.M. they helped me into our car and we left for Kalamazoo. First, I lay down in the back seat, but two blocks out of the hospital drive before we got on the Lodge that took up to I-94 West my husband stopped and I got in the front seat and tipped the seat back. I immediately fell asleep. I did wake up around Ann Arbor and told my husband to drive carefully as it was really raining. I woke up again when we got home at 8:30 P.M. They gave me Darvocet for pain and I took it as directed and it knocked me out. My Mom and youngest daughter came over to see me Friday afternoon and brought flowers. Our daughter came back over Saturday and did the laundry for me. Late Friday night was the last time I took the Darvocet as I wanted to get out of bed and couldn't as I was so sleepy. I didn't have any pain from the surgery which surprised me. I was instructed to wait for at least two days before removing the bandage. Sunday I got brave enough to take it off, and my husband helped. I almost fainted when it came off as my chest looked like a war zone. It was blue from the dye, yellow and bruised plus the incision was from my sternum to the outside of the nipple and my chest was flat. I was devastated as it looked like I had had a mastectomy. I had to put in stuffing to fill in the spot in my bra.

"When I went back to Detroit the next Thursday for my checkup, Dr. M., who examined me said that the tissue would come back and fill in some of the space. Dr. L. again apologized for how I looked as he knew I wasn't expecting that large of an incision as it was a partial mastectomy. But I told him I was glad I had him and his 37 years of experience for a surgeon as anyone else would probably have done a mastectomy and not tried to save anything. He was a very caring doctor and said I could have reconstructive surgery if I wanted. I told him "no, one surgery was enough." He told me I wouldn't be able to wear low-cut dresses anymore and I told him I didn't before, so it didn't matter. As they said, the breast tissue did fill in. It is slightly smaller than the right but I can wear regular undergarments with no padding and I look fine."

All surgeries do not lead to surprises such as Judith's discovery that the damage was worse than expected and that her chest "looked like a war zone." But I am impressed by her recovery from her initial shock.

Several of the other women mentioned surprises—usually unpleasant ones. From Jeannette: "My son came with me for my appointment. I was impressed by the care and attention given me. I can't say that I was afraid since I usually take things in stride. All went smoothly and when I awoke, I was in ICU. I was told that I had had a reaction to the dye that was used because it had sulfur in it and I am allergic to sulfur. I was surprised that this component was not known."

Another woman, Heidi, had a more serious surprise, but note how her emotional state became positive:

"The healing of the surgical wound was satisfactory, but I felt concerned about the drainage after a few days of surgery. I asked for a special appointment. I had developed hematoma which needed attention. Fortunately, there was no infection. Also, to my not-so-pleasant surprise, Dr. N. had to inform me that the pathologist's report now (after surgery) showed an invasive cancer of 1.2 cm. My surgery in February had been planned with a biopsy result of ductal carcinoma *in situ*, so that lymph nodes remained surgically untouched. This new development required an axillary lymph node removal. Due to the hematoma, this surgery had to be postponed for a few weeks. My numerous visits to Dr. N.'s office actually became pleasant, yes, they did. Dr. N. and his staff were extremely friendly; there was humor. They made me feel good and cared for.

"On May 12, I was scheduled for an axillary lymph node removal. Again, the team in the Preparation and Operating Room were kind, personal, and comforting. I remained calm. After waking up in the Recovery Room, I did not have any difficulties and was released."

Her doctor may have helped the recovery process "actually become pleasant," but we can also credit an internal strength of the woman herself.

D'Anna describes a very disturbing surprise in the outcome of her surgery:

"During my surgery, our pastors sat with my husband and parents at the hospital. I was cleared to go home about 10:30 P.M. On the way home in the car, I sat in the back seat with my mother and leaned on her shoulder. I asked how many lymph nodes they had had to remove. It was quiet for a while, and then my husband said, 'All of them.' I knew right then that I would have to have chemo. Dr. N. could tell that there was cancer in the sentinel node, so he removed 11 nodes, three of which were positive.

"I took the whole month of January off. At a birthday party, a neighbor asked me if I was pregnant. I actually wore a maternity top over the drainage bottles. Dr. N. had to drain some fluid, but I never felt the needle. I did, however, feel it when he pulled the drainage thing out! He told me to think of some place where I liked to go that was very relaxing, so I told him about our trips to the Outer Banks in North Carolina. After surgery, I thought I would never be able to lift my arm over my head again. I walked my hand up the wall every chance I got!"

Notice again the internal strength and courage that she summoned to work through this difficult situation. The support of D'Anna's family and her pastors were no doubt also very helpful.

But sometimes, as with Lucille, the surprise was something that the surgeons could address efficiently:

"In January '99 my mastectomy and reconstruction was performed at Henry Ford W. Bloomfield. I had two kinds of cancer—in situ and invasive, which hid behind white dots of calcium deposits. It was all very small and I avoided both chemo and radiation. Lucky me, only stuck with Tamoxifen."

Surprises are the exception. More often patients seemed to be taking their surgery in stride, as Heidi did:

"On February 17, 2003, I was scheduled for a total mastectomy of my left breast. Nurses and pre-anesthetist specialists prepared me for surgery. They were extremely kind, comforting, and professional. I did not feel any anxiety, no tranquilizer was necessary. Dr. N. visited and humored me. I was wheeled into the Operating Room, was kept warm, and fell asleep. After a few hours I woke up in the Recovery Room, felt a little queasy from the anesthesia, but not for a long time. At mid-afternoon I was released to go home."

How reassuring to hear her calm tone of voice. We hear the same tone in what Sonja says below:

"On January 24, 2000, I arrived at the hospital at 7:00 A.M. Had to go for the lymph scan in nuclear medicine. I was at the hospital from 7:00 A.M. until 6:00 P.M. that evening. There was no problem with the surgery. The sentinel node was cancer-free. That was good news. I was discharged at 6:00 P.M. Glad to be going home. Now I had to prepare for the radiation therapy, which I really didn't want to have. But I was getting much stronger in my faith."

Her concluding sentence speaks volumes. I don't think she is referring to her religious faith here, though she may be. I think she means her confidence—in her health care team, in her prospects for recovery, and in herself.

The "faith" of many of the women is strongly tied to self-confidence based on knowledge and the power that knowledge brings. Note how Beatrice describes her version of "faith":

"He wanted a needle biopsy—a simple process of inserting five needles into different sections and angles of the suspect area. At my request, I was allowed to watch on the TV monitor as each needle was carefully placed. It reminded one of the magician's box where the lady is placed inside as swords are thrust through the box at every angle. Of course she comes through unscathed. I knew I'd be fine and more specific information would be ours.

"At the first office visit with Dr. N. he described the sentinel node biopsy. He spoke of a partial mastectomy and not having to remove all the lymph nodes under the arm. I was very pleased to think that lymphedema would not be a problem in the future.

"The procedure to locate the sentinel node went smoothly. It was easy to watch the injected nuclear dye move around the tumor and up to the node where the ducts took the dye. Bone scans were made in early October with good results. Surgery quickly followed. The partial lumpectomy showed positive lymph nodes. I wanted to forego their removal. It seemed to me that with the removal of the infected area being followed by chemotherapy and then radiation, that more surgery was not necessary. I heard varying reactions from different doctors. It was up to me. After much investigation by our two daughters the decision was made to go back and remove the lymph nodes. This second surgery took place in early November. Along with removing the nodes, a port was put in place in my chest under the skin. This meant that instead of having numerous blood draws and other procedures where needles would be used in my veins, I had an 'open door' to those veins. It was painless and easier to use, making each medical visit smoother."

I am delighted here by her confidence ("I knew I'd be fine") and her clarity about who was responsible for the major medical decisions ("It was up to me."). Also impressive is her understanding of exactly what is going on. Her health care team had deeply involved her in the process of her treatment.

Sometimes patients were further energized in a positive way through their willingness to participate in research that would help other breast cancer patients. Isamay's experience is typical. Her involvement in research helped ease her experience, giving her the kind of power that helping others can provide:

"My lumpectomy was immediately scheduled. I had agreed to participate in the sentinel lymph node study (Dr. N.), hoping that whatever was to be learned would help someone in the future (and I have two granddaughters). On the appointed day, I reported for a mammogram and to nuclear medicine, then to surgery. Obviously I do not remember more than being prepped. The procedure, left lumpectomy with axillary lymph node dissection, was performed. I must say, however, that every person with whom I came in contact, was friendly, helpful, compassionate and caring—everyone!—receptionists, nurses, doctors—everyone!

"Sometime during the afternoon, I was discharged and returned home. I was sleepy, felt minimal discomfort and slept well that night. I do remember, however, our son's comment about my condition was that he thought I was 'spacey.' (Really!) I did not do much for a day or so, even though I felt fine."

Of course, there is no direct causal connection between her involvement in research and the relative ease of her recovery. On the other hand, there may be an important indirect connection through the attitude that reaches out in a constructive way. She is doing something rather than being a passive victim. Note the justified pride in Beatrice's voice:

"This surgery also included taking marrow samples. These would not affect my case. The marrow would be used to study cancer cases for the future, looking for what can be seen in the marrow that correlates with the disease. It's a good feeling to think you can add important pieces of future research."

Jackie had a similar kind of positive experience:

"I was asked to participate in an experiment to detect the Sentinel Lymph Node. This would save future breast cancer patients from having all of their lymph nodes removed. It would show the lymph nodes which were infected therefore saving the lymph nodes which were good. I believe they are now able to routinely use this procedure. The surgery went well. I had my left breast removed along with all sixteen of my lymph nodes. I came home the same day as my surgery. That is what I wanted. I had to let my three daughters know that I was all right. I really did not experience much pain from the operation."

Again, there is no direct causal link, but my intuition tells me that the positive attitude is important in shaping the experience, and the emotional experience shapes the recovery process. Julia continues in the same tone of voice: "Prior to my surgery I participated in a research study 'Molecular Markers in Breast Cancer Lymph Node Metastases.' This is very satisfying because I believe that shortly thereafter the sentinel lymph node became an accepted procedure."

Breast cancer patients also benefit tremendously from external support—from friends and family as well as health care professionals. We will see more of such support in later chapters, but I want to highlight a few examples more directly connected to the surgeries.

In the first example, written by Beverly, we see reassurance in a warm and humorous exchange between surgeon and patient at a crucial time: "The funniest moment was on the operating table. I was so cold and the nurse kept putting warm blankets on and as I was starting to feel a previous anesthesia (I guess in the IV) when Dear Dr. N. said he also felt cold and thought he would crawl in under the blankets—I wanted to say, 'you are welcome, but there's no room'—but could not mouth the words, so I guess I was ready to be put under."

And Lisa described parallel support between her doctor and her husband:

"Facing facts, I asked myself, what do I/we do about it? Can I handle surgery, radiation and other follow-up treatments? My doctors and oncology staff members helped with my unending questions and gave answers. Surgery was prescribed and I was fortunate to be assigned to, Dr. N., who performed a lumpectomy and sentinel biopsy. His kind gentle manner and soft comforting voice allayed any fears. Surgery day: I went from telling my husband, 'I love you, see you in a little while,' to waking up under a warm cozy blanket saying, 'Hi' to him and receiving discharge instructions. I believe my greatest concern of post surgery was dealing with lymphedema, fortunately there was none."

As I pointed out with earlier examples, the support from the medical staff here included answers to questions as well as the doctor's "kind gentle manner and soft comforting voice."

The comfort can even lead to an appreciation of the humor in a situation—if the attitude is right—as was the case with Rita:

"The morning of my surgery I had to go early to have dye injected. I guess so the doctor could find the lymph node specimen. The dye was not progressing as quickly as expected. By pure good luck my husband left the room and my daughter came in and was asked to massage my breast. My husband would have been so embarrassed to do this. The good doctor was in to see what the hold up was. My daughter and I laughed knowing how much longer it would have taken had my husband remained."

One of the most all-encompassing descriptions of support and comfort surrounding surgery came from Clara in this passage:

"October 6, 2000. We were at Henry Ford Hospital early. My daughter, son-in-law, and sister went with me. My daughter went with me to get the lymphatic imaging (radioactive dye) in the milk ducts so they could mark the skin where the surgeon should cut the lymph nodes. I asked her to hold my legs down, but the nurse did. Then we went back to the waiting room. A nurse brought me a warm blanket (I still have it). She also gave me sweet assurance everything was going to be all right. However, I signed a release, so if I died they would not be held responsible, because I couldn't have any healing meds since I was allergic. I really thought I was on my way to Heaven. This is my time to go, I told myself, and I was content, in good care, so much faith all around me, and such good people. I was taken to the preparation room. They let my daughter come in. Then Dr. N. came in. I told him I put him in the hands of the Lord, and prayed God would guide his hands and mind to do what had to be done. And knowing all the nurses, assistants and doctor, and how positive, gentle and pleasant they all were, I lost my fear and relaxed. My sister and son-in-law came in to see me. The anesthetist came in to put the IV in my arm. My family went to the waiting room. I was wheeled into the hall and about to go through the doors to surgery when I was out (lost consciousness). I didn't wake up till I was in the recovery room. That was about 12 hours from the time we arrived at the hospital. I had pain and was nauseated. The nurse put something in the IV bag and I was OK, but tired and weak. They put me in a wheel chair, and my family took me home, and the Lord healed me, and my family took care of me until I could manage alone, which was after my stitches and drainage bag were removed. I walked and did exercises and worked in my home to get back in shape.

"I think the warm blanket was so cozy and comfortable, it relaxed me, and I was relieved of my fears, and so it is in my memory mostly."

It was all working for Clara: family, the doctor, faith in the Lord, and the cozy warm blanket.

A boyfriend provided equally valuable support to Sharon through an uncomfortable procedure in a "cold and barren" setting:

"Dr. B. said it was a small cancer and should respond well to a lumpectomy with a sentinel node dissection. I was so glad to hear that I wouldn't lose several lymph nodes because I was very apprehensive of possible edema later in life.

"Inserting the dye to mark the first node was an uncomfortable procedure, but bearable with Dick by my side the whole time. I don't know if I would have had the courage to get through everything without Dick. Surgery was on November 1, 2001, and went well. I remember it being very cold and barren looking going through the hall to the OR. I asked the attendant if they were taking me to the morgue, reminding them that I wasn't dead yet. I was remarkably cheerful and upbeat the morning of surgery. Of course, Dick was there with me. The recovery wasn't too bad. Dick had to help me dress, as I couldn't lift my left arm. The doctor said there were clear margins and the cancer was small and I shouldn't require chemo. Dr. A., my oncologist, concurred and I started 30 radiation treatments after the wound was healed."

Her nervous sense of humor evident in her "morgue" comment also helped her through the experience.

And for Jennie it was neither family nor friend (nor warm blanket!), but a "special lady":

"The morning before my operation I had a sentinel lymph node dye test to see if any of my lymph nodes were affected and they were all clear and good. My husband and sister-in-law were in the room. My doctor was Dr. N. who did my test. With the lymph nodes clear, I did have my mastectomy and all went well.

"Before all of the testing, my two sisters and I had a conference with a special lady who also had breast cancer. She explained and told us about any help, who to call. What to expect after the operations, exercise, bras.

"So I had my mastectomy on November 10, 2000, and in January of 2001 I started my Nolvadex."

I suspect the "special lady" is employed by the hospital, but that really doesn't matter. Support is support. We all need it, we all can offer it, and we can take it wherever we can find it.

While the process of going through surgery is important, perhaps even more important is the outcome of the surgery. We don't want to confuse this outcome with the overall outcome of the recovery, something that may take years to evaluate.

Sometimes the surgical outcome is clear-cut, while sometimes it may be ambiguous. Beckie's was a rather straightforward report:

"The day of my surgery to remove my right breast started at 7:00 A.M. with a sentinel node biopsy that Dr. N. performed, nodes negative! From there to surgery and then on to recovery. Cancer caught early, stage 1, no chemo no radiation. I will go on Tamoxifen for 5 years."

And from Hardeep:

"The lumpectomy/mastectomy dilemma was very difficult. It took some time to decide. Once I had the lumpectomy, I felt as if I had gotten rid of something terrible, and that I had made some progress in treatment."

But often, as in Isamay's case, the outcome was more complex: "The following week I returned to the Surgeon (F.)—he had 'good news and bad news.' The good news was that the surgery went well—the bad news was that there were positive margins. So we scheduled another surgery. Same drill—all went well. About a week later, I developed a rash and was treated successfully." The patient took it all in stride and does what she has to do.

We see a similar ability to take what comes and do what is necessary in the following, written by Beckie: "Recovery was not all that bad. Sleeping was the worst part for me, as I could not lay flat so I slept on the couch. Feelings of being any less a woman? Not at all. I am still the same person. Having one breast is not an issue for me. If it becomes one there is always reconstructive surgery." Again, I sense here the results of good preparation by the medical team along with an inner strength that was there all along.

Preparation, however, can only do so much, as was the case with Susan:

"A lumpectomy is not an easy surgery. I have a slight problem in that I cannot take pain medication. It hurts my stomach and makes me vomit which pulls the stitches thus causing more pain than relieving it. Tylenol 3 is my new best friend. I was an outpatient and had to endure the ride home without the benefit of any pain medication. Believe me, I felt every bump in the road. I couldn't wait until my husband got back from the pharmacy with the Tylenol. At least it takes the edge off the pain."

Her "new best friend" may not be on a par with the friends and family that supported other women, but again, here is a person doing what she can to get through the difficult experience.

For a lucky few, like Francine, the recovery from surgery was relatively quick: "In January the surgery was performed. I felt sore the first day but only took one pain pill the day of surgery and that night. The recovery was easy."

For others like Marianne, however, there are problems that might have been prevented:

"Surgery was excellent, except for recovery room. They discharged me still obviously barely standing up and balancing. The night of my surgery day could have been a lot better had they kept me in the hospital or at least ordered an injectable antiemetic. I am a nurse and could have given it to myself or have someone give it to me. I was prescribed Compazine tablets I could not keep down."

Here the patient's knowledge came from her training and experience as a nurse rather than from what her medical team told her or her own efforts to self-educate. Unfortunately, her knowledge did not help her in this situation.

In the case of Sally Cole-Saul, her knowledge came from direct experience with her first breast cancer surgery:

"The first cancer surgery was a lumpectomy. When I went into the hospital I felt everyone was in a hurry and just wanted to get the procedure over. I knew it was very small, and told it would be just a few stitches. I was also told by the doctor there was only a small likelihood that it was cancer because of the size. I was initially relieved when the operation was over, but a few days later came the distressing news that the pathology was positive for cancer. I was not emotionally prepared for this bad news. The surgery was over but the decisions had only begun. In hindsight I now feel that I would have dealt much better with this had I had a second opinion and understood more of the ramifications.

"The second time I had done much more research, had acquired multiple inputs and opinions before making a final decision. I had decided the best option would be to have a sentinel lymph node biopsy performed with a double mastectomy and a tram flap. My husband, my best girlfriend and a healing-touch practitioner accompanied me right up until I went into surgery. Dr. N., my surgeon at Henry Ford spoke to me with a soft convincing voice to assure me everything would be fine. As I was being wheeled to the surgery and falling asleep under the anesthetic, my mind knew everything would be just what he said. I felt confident I was doing everything I could do to address this cancer and to prevent a re-occurrence of breast cancer."

It is my sincere hope that readers of this book can learn what Sally Cole-Saul had to learn from her first experience with cancer.

Surgery, including the recovery from surgery, is just the first part of the recovery process. Other unknowns lie ahead—chemotherapy and/or radiation for many, and then further fears that may never go away. As Alyce put it: "I guess the biggest fear I had was hoping the surgery would get all the cancer. It seems that happened, and now I pray for no recurrences." Her choice of words shows how hope and fear are intertwined, which is often the case as breast cancer survivors enter the next phase of their recovery.

6

CHEMOTHERAPY: "FEAR IS DIMINISHED WHEN YOU'RE AWARE"

For some breast cancer patients, the prospects of chemotherapy are almost as frightening as the disease itself. The powerful drugs involved lead to hair loss, weakness and fatigue, nausea, and a compromised immune system that makes people vulnerable to infections. There is a lot to worry about.

Despite these very real risks, cancer survivors have shown remarkable strength and courage in finding ways to confront chemotherapy and receive the benefits. I've found that although each story is different, we can see some common themes.

Many patients rely on support from nurses to get through what could have been an emotional ordeal. Hardeep said, "The first time I went for chemotherapy, I burst into uncontrollable tears there. The nurses were very supportive and assured me that they would take care of me." Beatrice found it valuable to give in to the weakness she felt:

"For me it was an easy experience. I was learning a great deal, such as the shots I gave myself of Nupogen that stimulates the bone marrow to make the white blood cells, so important in fighting infection. When the shots didn't bring the blood count up, we added an antibiotic. Everything being added and watched so carefully gave me full confidence that all would be well.

"The fatigue that occasionally took over reminded me of the similar feelings I had experienced many years ago during pregnancy. In giving in to the tiredness, instead of 'making a baby,' I was allowing my body to heal. We women often feel guilty if we read during the day. We think of the errands that need to be done, the laundry, the gardening, and the cooking. When you are pregnant with your first child is the easiest time to give into tiredness and feel good about doing so. When you are undergoing chemotherapy, again you have the chance to give in and enjoy the passage of time."

Isn't it surprising to find the word "enjoy" in a description of chemotherapy!

Beatrice even found a way—through her humor—to deal with the loss of her hair:

"Just a word about shaving off the hair. It's easier to shave it off rather than see it come off in your hands or on your bed pillows each day. My daughter did a smart thing. She set up a barber shop outside on the patio with her two young daughters in attendance. They could see that I was in no distress. In fact, we laughed a lot as we shaved away. They gathered up the hair to discard. Some of it flew off in different directions. A few days later I was pleased to show them a new bird's nest nearby that had my hair in it!

"I felt good and enjoyed the chance to try out different wigs. The American Cancer Society makes many new looks available. They have hats, tams, scarves, head pieces of all kinds with hair attached. I particularly enjoyed wearing a head band complete with brunette bangs and hair fluffed to the back of the neck. These are very reasonably priced. Their offices also have used and cleaned wigs and bras of every size, there for the taking.

"One day I could be a blond, the next—a red head; curly headed, pageboy cut or whatever I chose. I found that one of the most comfortable and striking ways to dress was to wear no wig—put on a scarf to match my clothes and a hat over the scarf. It can be a stunning look!"

Susan's response to her hair loss was similarly positive—a sign of her resiliently positive attitude:

"'Chemotherapy'—probably one of my worst fears. One always hears how awful chemotherapy is and, although it is certainly not pleasant, and there are some days that are worse than others, one really doesn't need to be as fearful of it as many people seem to be. The chemotherapy drugs have different side effects and there are medications your doctor can prescribe to ease most of the symptoms.

"One of the things that disturbed me most was the thought of losing my hair which was thick and always easy to manage and style. I thought to myself 'how vain can one be?' but your hair is part of your identity and it's a very common fear. It's not pleasant to lose your hair, but human beings can adjust to many things. The day my hair started falling out in large clumps, I had my hairdresser shave my head which helped me feel in control. My hair had always been very straight and when it started growing back it was very curly and you know what? I actually feel better with short curly hair. I've been told it'll grow in straight after a while but meantime, I'm having fun with it. I also haven't gone back to colouring it . . . and if it hadn't been for chemotherapy, I would NEVER have cut my hair this short, curled it and left it salt and pepper!!"

Susan went on to describe her experience in dealing with the consequences of her chemotherapy:

"I was very fortunate in being able to work from home during my chemo treatment, although I certainly could have gone into the office. This alleviated my commute to work downtown by subway and there certainly were some days when I felt very tired. At one stage my red blood cells fell so low, I had to have a blood transfusion and go onto a regime of injections and iron tablets to build up my red blood cells. I bounced back very quickly. Working was the best thing for me. It kept my mind busy and kept me involved in something other than myself. In fact, during the entire time I was having chemotherapy, there were only 5 days when I felt unable to work.

"I went back to work in the office one week after completing my last treatment of chemotherapy. I initially thought I'd work half-days till my energy returned to normal but I found that I could easily work full days from the first day back."

Of course, complications of one kind or another are to be expected. Note how Beatrice responded to what happened to her, starting with her moving to another state:

"My oncologist in Detroit found the oncologist in Florida who was dealing with the same protocol that I had started in Detroit. I met with the nurses who explained the drugs as they administered them into the port. The doctor checked me and the charts before they started and I reviewed the timing of the self medication, the antinausea drugs and the Nupogen shots. I felt comfortable with this new staff I was seeing. The clinical trial nurse, a nurse specialist, was assigned to me. She shared her cell phone number and told me to call anytime I felt the need."

And for a while she thought she was in the clear:

"January 21—the final chemotherapy. The pattern of the three weeks following the December 31 treatment appeared to be what was expected. The blood count kept going down. By January 7 the clinical trial nurse put me in quarantine: see no one, go nowhere. I was tired enough to give in and do nothing. By the third week I was feeling normal again."

But then:

"At the time of the last chemo treatment, the oncologist felt a lump under my left arm where the lymph nodes were removed. He made arrangements for an ultra sound immediately with a surgeon's visit the next day. The area under the arm became red, hot and larger, plus a fever of 101 degrees. The doctor ordered an antibiotic and I started taking the tablets immediately.

"When I saw the surgeon, he aspirated the lump. It had been diagnosed by the ultrasound to be a cyst. Soon the area of infection felt larger and 'heavier' under the arm. I went back to the surgeon who then took more fluid out and declared it to be cellulitis. Because I was still running a fever, I contacted the oncologist's office and spoke to another oncologist—mine was not available. This doctor said to just 'wait and see what happens.' The fever registered only 100.2 degrees, but I realized that my immune system was compromised by the recent chemo. This was four days after the last treatment, so disregarding this 'wait and see' attitude, I called the surgeon who had aspirated the area. I wanted his advice about going to the hospital to get a blood draw and if the white count was low—to get an IV in the hospital.

"He agreed that I should get to the hospital, but since this wasn't a surgical problem, admittance should be under the oncologist's name. He strongly encouraged me to call my oncologist quickly. I called and reported my concerns to the doctor who said that she'd call the hospital to order the blood draws.

"After arriving at the hospital through emergency, I found that no request had come from the oncologist. It was the ER physician who felt strongly that I should be admitted, got the blood draws and began the antibiotic IV while still in emergency.

"When I met the female oncologist who was filling in over the weekend for my doctor, she thought I had acted correctly, even though she had given no support when asked for it. She was to order Nupogen when I saw her. She didn't do this either. So I used the vial my husband brought from home. I called the Michigan oncologist who told me not to wait—'Take the Nupogen now.' This all took place in the hospital over the weekend. By Monday cramping, diarrhea and retching began, lasting throughout the night and the following day. Thank goodness, my own oncologist was back and he made arrangements for the infectious disease doctor to see me. The surgeon was to visit as well.

"I thought that the rough time was because of the IV antibiotics making me ill. The oncologist explained that it was the cumulative effects of the chemo treatments. For the first time, I began to understand how a cancer patient feels when the body rebels. Fortunately, this was the only bad time I had. I know now how patients' systems can be so compromised, they can hardly get through it. How lucky to have had these bad hours in the hospital rather than at home. Here I had the help of the nursing staff who were wonderful. I didn't want my husband to have to deal with these explosions of bodily functions. Knowing what causes this makes the process bearable. Fear is diminished when you're aware of *why* things happen.

"The next days were easier. Pain was kept to a minimum and I felt stronger although talking was still an effort. The IV antibiotics were administered around the clock, and when the blood counts came up, I was released from the hospital. I could then go to the infectious disease doctor's office daily to manage the cellulitis.

"Aspiration of the area under the arm took place again—another 60 milliliters (third time). The culture showed no malignant cells. Naturally I felt better overall and began to eat again. The realization that we are all responsible for ourselves was strong after this experience. Dealing with inadequate doctors happens. Reaching out to others makes decisions easier. It also restores a sense of power.

"By the end of the week I was feeling much better even though the nail on my big toe came off due to the chemo. But so had my eyebrows and most of the eyelashes. Make up can do wonders, and I was ready to go home.

"While still in the hospital, my daughter from Detroit arrived for a quick visit. I was now pretty good, so I made a 'dummy' in the bed with pillows and one of my wigs—all curled up under the covers. It looked like a wasted body in a fetal position. My husband and daughter arrived from the airport. As they walked down the hospital corridor, I followed them in back. Their reaction to the figure in the bed was great. I let them know I was behind them. Then we all laughed and carried on like normal. At that point a nurse entered and went right to the dummy to take my vital signs. She had a pretty strong reaction too—Laughter is such a positive force!

"The surgeon returned that evening—aspirated for the fourth time—another 60 milliliters. This continued for another 12 aspirations in the surgeon's office plus daily visits to the infectious disease doctor for IV antibiotics.

"So what caused the cellulitis? Could it have been the tiny scratch I got on my arm when I was pruning the bougainvillea? This I know and will gladly pass on—care of the skin surface is a must when those lymph nodes are removed. Rubber gloves come in handy. Careful manicures are important. Cuts of any kind, whether from preparing food or opening a letter, need to be tended to properly.

"The ongoing aspirations were frustrating but not painful. The ongoing visits to the infectious disease doctor made me feel like a patient forever. But this too finally came to an end."

Just notice all of the signs of Beatrice's attitude: when she saw a problem, she addressed it, whether it was by involving another doctor or applying makeup! She armed herself with knowledge to help her make good choices and to keep fear at bay. She was aware that the experience of chemotherapy would end. And she never lost her sense of humor. Also note how she described the process of giving herself shots for 3 months:

"Fortunately a special protocol was offered to me. It was a fairly new study that combines the drugs needed plus a drug called Taxotere. The best part— I needed to take these drugs for only three months instead of the normal 6 months of chemotherapy. No matter how hard the drugs may be, it's much easier to handle anything when it's for only three months. Shots of Nupogen were the answer to help bring back the blood levels. How easy it is to take shots when you're the one giving them to yourself!"

"Fortunately," she said, and "the best part," and "how easy." Chemotherapy may not have seemed so easy at the time, but here is another lesson: over time, the right attitude can help shape the nature of your experience.

Another woman, Eve, experienced a different complication:

"Everything sounded very simple, but I had a big problem. After my second chemotherapy I got a rash and the dermatologist told me that I am allergic to the chemotherapy. Dr. S. told me that I had two options and both were risky.

"The first option: I can jump to Taxol maybe I will tolerate it better but my treatment will not be complete, so I take risks. Second, I can have Benadryl and other antiallergic medicines with my chemotherapy and swallow some antihistamines, but if we fail to control the rash it will be risky. I decided to go on with my chemotherapy because I wanted to get cured. I knew that the chemotherapy was important for me so I took the risks of the antihistamines. The antihistamines elevated my blood sugar, which I tried to reduce with a healthy diet.

"For me as a patient the most important thing was a good attitude, positive thinking and the spiritual power that my belief in God and my family gave me. The best doctors are not able to do the job if we as patients don't help ourselves with understanding the problems and trying to have a good attitude. We have to care and to take everything very seriously because cancer is a difficult and tricky illness. I tried to continue my life as usual. I did my housework every day. I saw my friends, and we went to movies, concerts, and museums maybe more than usual perhaps to prove to myself that I was able to do so. All this between the treatments. I love the saying, 'Look good, feel good.'

"I always try my best and it helps. However, spiritual power and goodwill are not enough. I was lucky that my blood tests were good and I could finish my chemotherapy in 6 months. Dr. S. told me that I have to see him every 3 months the first year and then every 6 months for check ups. I appreciate everything he did for me. He was always very understanding with a lot of good will and he helped me more than I can tell. I felt safe with Dr. S., and I am grateful for everything he has done for me, but I was a good patient too. I did all my check ups, all my blood tests every week and everything showed that my body was recovering before the next treatment. I finished my chemotherapy on 5/16/2000."

She said, "if *we* fail to control the rash," showing her active involvement with her health care team in the process of her recovery. Eve was fully aware of the importance of God, family, and doctors, but she was not at all a passive recipient of help from those sources. She did her part.

I do not want to give the impression that complications from chemotherapy are the rule. Yvonne's description is perhaps more typical:

"My chemotherapy treatment, with the help of all the wonderful drugs on the market, was not so bad. The best way I can describe how I felt was that it was like a very bad hangover, but the next day it was better, much better, and I looked at it as 'one treatment down, only—more to go.' I will tell you though it was a happy day when I walked out of that chemotherapy room for the last time."

And Alyce's description:

"Fortunately, I had mild chemo, but it did play havoc occasionally. Not too often. One of my most memorable experiences was the kindness and sympathy the nurses showed, not only me, but my husband as well. He always accompanied me when I had chemo."

The woman identified as Judith in earlier chapters also reported:

"The following week I meet with Dr. A. at the Dearborn site regarding chemo treatments. Because of my age, the grade and size of the tumor, he said it was up to me if I wanted to go through chemo. He said it would increase my longevity by 3 percent. I decided I would be able to live to 103 instead of 100 so I said I wanted to have it. On October 23 I had my first treatment which went well except for the dreaded IV they had to use. I had treatments the third and fourth Wednesday of each month through December at Dearborn. We have a place in Florida which we are at from January 1 to April 15 every year, and we really wanted to go to Florida for the winter. Dr. A. said that was no problem as they had a lot of patients that continued their treatments there. So I made some calls and found an excellent facility at Venice Oncology in Venice

FL near our home. I started there in January and finished my treatments there. They had a blood testing machine that they could prick your finger and tell in a matter of minutes if the counts were where they should be for another treatment. Also, they used the butterfly apparatus in the vein and inserted the chemo there. It was a 5- to 10-minute operation and no IVs. Dr. L. was very supportive and she answered all the questions I had at the end of March as my next appointment with Dr. A. wasn't until April 10.

"I did really well with the chemo. I didn't get nauseated but did lie down a lot as I was exceptionally tired. I didn't lose all my hair but it did get really thin. I was able to get a nice wig in Sarasota FL which I wore when I went out. My hair has since come in thicker but unfortunately still gray."

Judith skipped quickly over the negatives ("the dreaded IV") and, like Beatrice, was able to keep her sense of humor.

D'Anna, whom we met in Chapter 2, showed some of the same pragmatic problem-solving attitude we have seen in other women:

"Another 'Brownie mom' told me I should think about getting a port. I am so thankful I did! It made getting chemo and blood tests so much easier. We decided to go on a study, and I ended up in the control arm that my oncologist said he would recommend if I didn't want to go on the study. I had four treatments of Adriamycin and Cytoxan, followed by four treatments of Taxol. The Taxol was the worst, which wasn't saying much, because I was never sick. I never even felt the least bit nauseated.

"My daughter's Brownie troop provided dinner on the night before each of the eight chemo treatments. Even though I was not the primary cook in the family, it was much appreciated. It was so nice that my husband didn't have to worry about that in addition to everything else.

"Two weeks to the day after my first treatment my hair started falling out. I was amazed at how much hair I had. It kept coming out and coming out and coming out and it still looked like I had a full head of hair! I told someone at work that my hair had started falling out and he said, 'At least yours will grow back in.' So I decided that maybe I shouldn't mention it to guys who were bald! On Saturday night, I stood under the shower and let the water knock out as much hair as it could. I kept picking the hair off the drain and I saved all that hair, to compare with my new hair when it grew back in. My parents came down the next day and we shaved my head. I was so glad my hair had started falling out because it meant that the chemo was doing at least one thing I had been told about! I had my wig, and I wore it to work. Most people couldn't tell that it was a wig. I got a lot of compliments about it. But as soon as I got out in the car to go home, off it came.

"My husband liked to say that 'Henry Ford Hospital didn't let you get sick.' I had antinausea pills, but they emphasized that there were other ones we could try if those didn't work. I took one the night after my first chemo, just because I wanted to prevent any nausea, but that was the only one I ever took. I heard the chemo nurses 'bawl' patients out because they hadn't called them when the pills didn't work.

"The Taxol caused the most 'problems.' I took the pre-Taxol pills and the nurse sat and watched me for about 5 minutes after she started the IV for the first time. Then she went back about her business. Soon though, I felt very hot and started having trouble breathing. I asked (no one in particular) if my face was red. Everyone looked up at me and the nurse quickly stopped the IV. She started a different IV and told me that I would have to have this before each Taxol treatment. I got mouth sores and went to Dr. A. to see what he could do about them. He gave me a prescription for 'Magic Mouthwash,' something the oncologists and pharmacy had come up with. He told me I had to take the prescription to a HFH pharmacy because no one else would know what it was! It worked pretty well! I had one of my treatments delayed due to a low white count. So then I had to give myself shots to help keep the counts up.

"I had treatments on the Thursday before Easter, and on the Thursday before my youngest brother's wedding, but I didn't have to miss either one! I felt fine! My hair started growing back during the Taxol treatments, and I started to wear a pink 'Race for the Cure' cap. Following a quickie vacation to the UP [Michigan's Upper Peninsula], I began radiation treatments which lasted until September 25, 2000."

I love the way she described how she responded to the potentially devastating loss of her hair.

Emotions, simply put, are a significant feature of the disease. Hardeep reported, "Many ups and downs during treatments—depression, anxiety, and sometimes OK." She went on to note, "I mostly kept up my regular activities during treatment. I used to rest a lot. And I would often feel very depressed."

It's easy to say one should keep a positive attitude, but sometimes despite your best efforts you get worn down. Jackie's story illustrated this:

"Next step was back to see Dr. V. to get the pathology report and to have my drain removed. The pathology report was not as good as I had hoped for. The cancer had traveled to three of my sixteen lymph nodes. This meant I would have to have six months of aggressive chemotherapy. At this time, I was referred to my oncologist, Dr. A. He also is a very caring person who always had time to answer every question that I had. My first visit he explained in detail what chemotherapy I would be receiving. I believe it consisted of four rounds of Adriamycin and Cytoxan and three rounds of Taxotere. He recommended I have a port installed to administer the chemotherapy through, as it can be very hard on your veins. I had the port installed and it proved to be the best thing I could have done. Receiving the chemo through the port was painless and all of my blood draws were taken from the port.

"I guess the worst feeling for me was that I felt I had no control over my life anymore. When my hair started falling out after my second chemo treatment I took control and let my thirteen-year-old daughter practice her hair-cutting skills and then had my husband buzz the rest off. To me that was much better than watching it fall out in handfuls day after day.

"Chemotherapy was very hard on me. I was not able to work for about seven months. Some days I felt so weak I could hardly get out of bed. I never really felt the why me scenarios as I was thankful it was not happening to someone else I loved. I kept a very positive attitude through this whole ordeal. Even with a positive attitude there were some days when I would have to have a good cry. I gained about thirty pounds and was very puffy looking. I had not one hair left on my body anywhere. It changed my appearance so much that the people I had known for years would walk right by not knowing it was me."

The sense of the loss of control that she described is important, and a number of women found some way to regain a feeling of control—from removing your own hair rather than watching it fall out, to deciding to participate in a research study to help battle the disease itself, to learning all you can about your disease so you can make the best choices for you.

Sometimes the choice is not to have chemotherapy, as Susan explained:

"Dr. D. wanted me to have chemotherapy. My tumor was one centimeter which is on the fence size wise for radiation and chemotherapy or just radiation. Both rounds would be followed by five years of Tamoxifen. I did not want chemotherapy and told Dr. N. I asked him if it were his wife or daughter what he would recommend. He said, 'Radiation and Tamoxifen.' That's what I did and I'm glad my fifth year of Tamoxifen is over. I am a moody person and menopausal. I have also had brain surgery. I didn't need a new drug introduced into my system to make me more emotional than I already am. Tamoxifen makes you weepy and crazy. These magnifications I do not need. Now I'm back to my old self. I'm just moody and menopausal but I'm fun!"

And sometimes, as in Roxanne's remarkable story, the decision to pursue chemotherapy comes from a complex set of sources and circumstances:

"I dealt well with the surgery. I was depressed but handled things well. After the surgery, I was given an appointment with Dr. A. He sent me to have other exams, CT scan, bone scan, and an electrocardiogram. The results came back negative and all well. I thought it was over. But then he tells me I have to have 'chemo.' I began to cry and told him, 'No.' He proceeded to explain why I should. He said I was healthy and that I would be able to withstand the treatment. He didn't say much, but he did have a lot of patience talking to me.

"I was more afraid of the treatment than of dying. Dr. A. sent me to see a psychologist. I only saw this woman twice and never returned. Dr. A. wanted to know why. I told him, 'She is going back all the way to my childhood!' I didn't need help with my childhood; I needed help to deal with this terrible disease, *now*!! I told Dr. A. that she would not be able to bring my breast back (meaning, she could not put things the way they were). I began to read books from a friend of mine who is a cancer survivor too. I found a great comfort and understanding in these books.

"I was given a few days to reconsider and give Dr. A. an answer regarding my decision to have chemotherapy. One evening, I went home and sat in my living room sofa alone. I grabbed my Bible and asked God to help me make a decision whether I should have this treatment. I asked him for a sign and I fell asleep on my sofa. I had an incredible dream that night. I dreamed that an Archbishop (I am Catholic) came to my apartment. I woke up and looked at the bottom of my door and jumped out of the sofa and went directly and opened the door. The archbishop was coming in through the wall. I stopped him and asked him to come in through the door. He came out of the wall and came in through the door. He was always smiling, and chanting a hymn. He came in and I could see his face very clearly, his blue eyes, and he was wearing a hat typical of an archbishop. I kissed his hand and I could feel the warmth. He began to walk towards my sofa when he suddenly stopped and extended his arm, spreading his hand and pointing it at me. With a great smile he said to me, 'Don't worry. Everything is going to be all right.' And he kept repeating those words over and over until I woke up. I told my best friend about this incredible dream. Her opinion was that I had a vision and in this vision a message I had asked God to give me.

"I began chemotherapy on October 31, 1999. I felt weird that morning, but I did go from the therapy to work. The day after the treatment I felt terrible—my stomach ached, nausea, etc. The good thing was that I didn't have to go to work the next day. I did have to go for the Nupogen shot to the hospital for the next 10 days. My insurance did not cover the shots. I didn't have prescription coverage. Basically, I felt really sick the first eight days.

"My biggest fear was not being able to sustain myself during the intensified treatment when I had to recuperate by rebuilding my defenses and could not work. I had no funds. I had a talk with God. 'You want me to do this treatment, you sent me a message that it was going to be all right then? . . . You are going to take care of this money issue and I am not going to worry about it.' I had no idea where the money was going to come from. A friend of mine showed up at my doorstep and handed me a check for $1,300 and said, 'Pay me when you can. I just want you to get well, and don't worry about money.' That very moment, I heard (I am very spiritual) a voice that said, 'You will have the money to pay her back.' (I had dreams before where I see an angel, with a very soft voice and it's not a person, it's a light, in the shape of a cross and it just waves around and warns me of something to come. You can laugh all you want or think that I am crazy, but I know this is true.) I had two more dreams where I saw myself with a wig. (I had not bought the wig yet! And in the dream the wig was exactly like the one I bought.) I didn't realize until after I bought it! In my dream I am happy and getting back to my life. I see the sunshine from spring and the trees budding."

Roxanne drew upon a wide array of resources to get her through the experience: the doctors, her family, God, dreams, a generous friend, and ultimately her own intuition. Whatever works for you!

7

RADIATION: "YOUR PERSONAL BATTERY RUNS WAY LOW"

Although radiation is not generally as frightening as chemotherapy, it can have its difficulties. Radiation oncology centers are not as easily available as chemotherapy suites/offices; the machines that deliver the radiation are expensive and, in Michigan at least, the numbers of centers approved for this highly specialized form of cancer treatment are strictly controlled by the state government. Most patients have to travel quite large distances to the nearest radiation oncology center, adding to the difficulties they have already experienced with surgery and chemotherapy. The radiation is directed at the diseased breast by carefully calculated movement of large radiation sources that move around the patient. Some patients fear the inevitable loneliness and uncertainty of being alone in a lead-lined room with a large machine, communicating with the radiation technologist by microphones and speakers. The treatment is delivered quickly, usually in about 5 minutes per treatment, and one doesn't feel anything directly. However, the average treatment is given daily, Monday through Friday, usually lasting 6 weeks. Scheduling these treatments is often accommodated quite easily to adjust to the patient's needs. Most women tend to coordinate their radiation treatments with their work and social schedules. The difficulty is adjusting to the daily routine of a fairly lengthy treatment.

Many women fear radiation since it has been played up in our minds by the association with atomic bomb blasts and the particularly scary events of the Chernobyl disaster, the Three Mile Island nuclear leak, and the mysterious murder of a Russian spy. Some women had seen bad effects of radiation in relatives or friends treated with this modality in earlier years, when modern technology was not as well developed. The bad effects in the past were unfortunately all too visible, in the form of massively swollen arms. Other bad side effects, seen many years ago, were dramatically reported to relatives and friends and consisted of bad burns. The unfortunate victims of these side effects often spent years in pain and were disfigured. Many other bad effects of radiation, no longer seen, may be remembered by older women and can produce considerable fear.

The most common acute side effect of radiation in the modern era is slight weakness and malaise, usually seen about 2–3 weeks after starting treatment in the radiation department. The stories in this chapter describe the feelings well. Patients who sunburn easily may have mild skin burns, usually toward the end of the treatments, and often managed quite easily with mild skin lotions, creams, or ointments. These side effects are certainly not universal and most people notice hardly any ill events. But, even those that had some ill effects from their radiation showed great strength and resourcefulness in overcoming those difficulties, relying on the expertise of health care professionals, support from family and friends, and their own internal sources of resilience.

First, let's hear Elaine walk us through her experience in radiation:

"My next appointment was with the Radiation doctor (Dr. G.) who suggested that I have more surgery to remove marginal tissue before treatments started. After returning to my surgeon and discussing the matter, I decided to go for additional surgery. This was performed on April 10. The third surgery confirmed that all the surrounding tissue was free of cancer. What a relief! After a 2-week rest for healing to take place the radiation treatments began. The first session is called a pretreatment visit. This is also referred to as a "simulation" because the patient goes through all the steps of treatment except receiving the radiation. On this visit x-rays are taken and measurements done to pinpoint the exact treatment area.

"As a patient I was provided with detailed written information on everything that happens during this experience. The radiation therapists do their best to make you comfortable and relaxed for each treatment. And the radiation doctor consults with you on a weekly basis. On each visit nurse K. takes your temperature and blood pressure and answers any questions you may have. Also, you receive phone numbers to call in case you have any other questions. The hospital has a cancer library on the premises where you can interact with other people with cancer and their families in a support group. This is an online patient-to-patient service located in the Patient Care area. The center also has a Web site where you will find answers to all of your questions.

"After the initial pretreatment visit, I was scheduled for my weekly radiation treatments. There is a separate entrance at the hospital for Radiation and Oncology patients. We are even provided with close-in parking spaces. When you enter the building the first person you see is Diane at the receptionist desk. Once you have told her your name she remembers you when you come again. She is pleasant and cheerful. Next, you go to a small changing room where you are provided with a gown and robe. They are in a large plastic bag with your name on. You will use it each time you come for a treatment. Outside of the changing room are two chairs where you can sit and wait for your appointment. The timing is excellent. You do not have to wait very long for your scheduled time. Soon a radiation therapist greets you by name and chats with you to ease any nervousness, and takes you into the treatment room. You get up on a table, are helped into the exact position needed, marks are placed on your body to pinpoint the area to be treated. The amount of radiation is determined by your doctors and is carefully monitored. When you are comfortable on the table, the therapist explains how the procedure works and the process begins. Kim, Susan, Sally, and Paula were my therapists and did a marvelous job of making the situation easy for me.

"The treatment itself is painless. You hear the whirring of the machine as it zaps the exact location on your body where radiation is needed. In a few minutes the therapists are next to the table and ready to assist you as you get up and off the machine. You then go to the changing room and get dressed leaving your hospital gown in your own special plastic bag. As you pass by the receptionist desk on your way out of the building S.S. wishes you a good day."

I am struck here by how personal Elaine's experience is. She is on a first-name basis with her radiation therapists. And as she tells her story, she is connecting with "you," the readers of this book. While the details of the procedure will of course vary from hospital to hospital, the simple fact is that radiation, like every part of the breast cancer experience, is a deeply personal experience from start to finish—even though it involves the science of tumor biology, biochemistry, pharmacology, and physics.

One thing that makes it so personal is the individual way that each breast cancer patient responds to each stage of her treatment. Beatrice, who we got to know in Chapter 5, continued through radiation therapy with her wonderfully positive attitude:

"The radiation process followed and was fascinating. Daily visits were combined with friends to shop or to lunch or to just visit. So the 8 weeks went by. It was longer because they were also radiating part of my neck. I didn't know this so the cream used wasn't applied to that area. The burn took some time to heal. We live and learn!"

Isamay had a similarly positive experience, attributing her success to her "A-Team":

"I met with my medical oncologist (Dr. C. Main Campus), as well as my radiation oncologist (Dr. G., West Bloomfield Campus). She suggested I prepare my skin for the radiation with lotion. The next week, I began my daily trek to West Bloomfield for my radiation treatments (25 plus 8 boosts). What a staff! I called them my A-Team—they were super! How fortunate for me—I did not experience the fatigue usually associated with the radiation therapy. We maintained a pretty normal life, even played some golf. Chemotherapy was not prescribed for me."

And for Judith, another relatively easy time with radiation:

"On April 28, I started my radiation at the West Michigan Cancer Center in Kalamazoo, Michigan. They did the simulation first and then I went in every weekday for 6 weeks for treatment. Toward the end they did a CT scan and did the final pattern for the boost. I didn't have any problems with the radiation as far as burning. I used the creams they gave me, faithfully. I was a little more tired than usual. But I made it through. I was even able to skip one day of treatments in order to go on a bus trip with the local Genealogical Society to do research. That was a bright stop as genealogy is my hobby and it gave me a better outlook on what was going on."

Her story is matched by Eve's:

"The radiation period was a piece of cake after the chemotherapy. I was told that the side effects of the radiation therapy are in long term so it was not bad for the moment. My breast got burnt a little bit. Dr. W., Radiation Oncology, checked me every week and gave me cream to ease the pain of the burn to my breast. It was not so bad. My first radiation was on 7/18/2000 and I finished on 8/5/2000. I had 34 radiation treatments."

And from Francine: "The pathology report showed a small cancer, which had not invaded the lymph nodes. My follow-up treatment involved taking Tamoxifen daily and 6 weeks of radiation once the incision healed. The radiation treatment was painless and other than some red skin and a little tiredness I didn't alter my life at all."

And from Yvonne: "Next was radiation therapy and again it was not a bad experience at all. Very few side effects."

From Marianne: "Radiologist and most techs were excellent."

From Roxanne: "Radiation was uneventful. I didn't burn severely. I didn't like the doctor and I was happy it was over. It did make me feel weak."

And from Ethel: "There were 35 radiation treatments, which did not make me sick and my energy levels remained near normal. I continued with my many political, union, and community activities. My strength came from within myself."

Some reported taking their treatment and their work schedules in stride. Margaret wrote, "I went for treatments then drove to work on my regular shift—in office." And Marianne said, "I was working part-time during my radiation treatments. Not the chemo." They did not point out what pain or fatigue they may have struggled with.

And Susan reported a similar response to radiation: "I had radiation after chemotherapy. I was lucky in that the hospital I was treated at is a 10-minute walk from my office, so I'd work a full day, schedule my radiation appointments after work and then hop on the subway to go home. I found radiation very easy and didn't have any side effects, other than a 'tanned look' in the radiated area, which faded back to my normal skin tone a few months after treatment was completed. My energy level was normal and I didn't feel tired at all."

Radiation treatment does not always go so smoothly, however. Jeannette stated bluntly:

"The radiation was the worst part of the treatment. I had quite a burn from it. I am in my fifth year since the surgery and am fine. I am 85 and not worried of a reoccurrence. In fact, I am surprised to be called a 'cancer patient.' Radiation went well 'til the end, when I received 2/3 degree burns that lasted a *long* time."

And Linda P., who we met in Chapter 2, described her difficult experience:

"My surgery went well. I had a sentinel node procedure with just a few tumors in the lymph node. I opted not to go with chemo. My radiation therapy started 6 weeks after surgery. The first few weeks weren't bad, but as it progressed I got more and more tired and the treated area was getting burned, which was painful, and since my job involved working with my hands I was unable to work during the last stages of radiation and through the healing process."

Pain and fatigue are not unusual. "The radiation made me tired," Georgina said, speaking for many. The question is what to do about the pain and fatigue. Here is D'Anna's response:

"Because of my fair skin, my radiation oncologist was worried about burns and blistering. I had a nice square 'sunburn' on my right breast, but that is all. It was a little red and itchy, but I slathered on the Aquaphor they gave me and tried not to scratch it too much!"

Lotion is a simple and direct solution. Lisa's approach was a bit more complex:

"Since the oncology team was in charge of my medical care I decided to handle my part with help from the 5 F's: Faith, Family, Friends, Focus, and Future. The first three I was certain I could count on; the fourth and fifth were focus on the future. The future was, besides my husband's care, our first grandchild was due, so I started counting the days until my son called to say, 'It's a boy.' Pictures via the Internet sent by grandson Lane's O.B. helped to shorten the distance between here and Denver, Colorado. During this time I was also counting the days of my radiation treatments and before long 33 had gone by. Though somewhat limited by fatigue following surgery and during radiation, I managed to drive myself to all my treatments, care for my husband, and do a few routine household chores for short periods of time. I was determined cancer was not going to control me or my life."

Several breast cancer survivors mentioned the 5 F's, which contribute to the emotional and psychological components of survival that lotion alone cannot touch. And several, like Sharon, reflected the importance of retaining the feeling of control:

"I started 30 radiation treatments after the wound was healed. I didn't burn or get particularly uncomfortable. I never missed a weight training session at Bally's or curtailed any activities. I felt a little glitch in my throat after a treatment but went about my business. I could have gone to work but I was laid off, nothing to do with the cancer. I still did my daily body toning routine and every other day weight lifting at Bally's."

Sally Cole-Saul also continued her routine as best she could:

"I worked during the entire period of the radiation. Perhaps I was a little tired from the radiation. I do not feel that my work was impacted in any significant way, but I was always conscious of my fears about the radiation (and of course, the cancer.)"

Her lingering fears are not at all surprising. She continued:

"I found Radiation too scary; I was tattooed so the radiologists could line up the same location each time. My fear was about what else will the radiation might damage (my skin, my lungs, etc.). My other concern was whether it would really do what it was intended to do."

Where some women, like Beatrice, saw their recovery process as an opportunity to get needed rest, others persisted in doing what was most important in their lives. We saw this when me met Sally Sawyer back in Chapter 5.

Sonja found her primary source of resilience in her faith:

"My radiation treatments began February 18 and ended April 26. There was no problem with my therapy. My husband was very faithful in driving me to the hospital every day. He was with me every day until the end of my therapy. I am a Christian, and I believe the prayers of my pastor, church, family, friends, and my faith helped to get me through my crisis. The only fear I had was having the radiation therapy. Then I prayed and asked God to take control of my fear. For I knew God had not given me the spirit of fear, but of power and of love and of a sound mind."

She sees her faith working through her family and friends, feeding her own internal strength.

On the other hand, Margaret found her strength in knowledge: "Radiation and chemo therapists were very clear with explanations of the hows, whys, etc., keeping close tabs on me all during treatments. This helped me a great deal—both physically and emotionally."

Others found strength by solving the practical problems associated with their treatment, as Lizabeth shows:

"I worked throughout my cancer treatments. Radiation treatments, since they were every day, had the biggest impact on my schedule. I participated in a clinical trial to protect my skin and painted on some material an hour before any radiation appointment. With nothing better to do I would walk on the treadmill every day before the appointment. I would then get dressed, drive the few miles to the clinic, get undressed, get radiation, and then get dressed again. After doing that a few times, I figured out that if I did not get dressed before leaving for the clinic I could save time. I just put on pants, threw on a coat and took my shirt with me. I could be in and out of radiation in a few minutes and be on my way to work."

The full emotional complexity of radiation therapy becomes clear in the story of Susan W.'s experience, which reveals the emotional ups and downs that are all too common:

"When we returned from Hawaii I went back to work. I also started my $6^1/2$ weeks of radiation. The radiation was postponed for the Hawaii trip. My job hours were a split shift 9 A.M. to 11 A.M., and I would return for 4 P.M. until 9 P.M. closing. My radiation treatments were every weekday Monday to Friday at 11:30 A.M. I was asked to be in a double blind study for medication that might help with radiation burn. Dr. G. asked me to sign up and I immediately did so. After all, I had to have the treatments anyway and this might help someone in the future. Before the surgery, I had been washing with expensive moisturizing soaps from health food stores. I read in one of the many books on breast cancer I had purchased that it was a good idea to prepare your skin before the surgery and especially before, during, and after radiation. One had shea butter in it and another had coconut oil, avocado, and other natural ingredients. I was still using them along with moisturizing creams and lotions. During and after radiation I found Aquaphor and Elta balms especially good. You have to use a lot and I cut a white T-shirt to use as dressing. Use a towel to protect bedding. The balm spot came off my knit PJ's just fine.

"The capsules were given to me for the study. You didn't know if you were given the real medicine or not. One half hour before your radiation time you were to break open the capsule mix with 1/2 cup water and add food color (your choice of color). You would smear this concoction from shoulder to mid chest to ribs, of course including your breast. Every day I would bring my little kit to work. It consisted of a measuring cup, a small bowl, cotton balls, food color, and the capsule for that day. I soon learned to condense my kit to a small Tupperware cup of blue water that I would just add the capsule to. My food color choice was blue. About 45 minutes before my appointment I would run to the bathroom at work and strip off my top and bra and mix this stuff and smear it on. I would then dry my breast under the hand dryer so I could get dressed and leave for my appointment. I did this 5 days a week for $6^1/_2$ weeks. I thought a blue boob would be funny. Actually, I want to go bright yellow so on the last day of radiation I could make a smiley face boob. You have to look for the fun side of things. I've been through enough to know that.

"I think I got the real medication in the study because I hardly burned at all. It was like a bad sunburn at its worst point. When I got the boost twice I had some tiny blisters right after. They were gone by the next morning. That might be a testament to the creams and lotions and soaps too. As you wait for your turn for radiation it struck me that age was not a determining factor. Of the four ladies waiting, we were each decades apart, ranging from 70 to 30 years old. One lady had to stop her radiation because her burns were so bad. I felt lucky.

"One thing about radiation, along about the fourth week your personal battery runs way low. The technicians in radiation warned me it would be cumulative and it would hit me the third or fourth week. Sure enough, like a car running on fumes I thought I'd have to pull over soon to fill up my tank before I could go on. There was nothing to renew my energy. Unfortunately, I had to go back to work and deal with the kind of ladies that send back water in a restaurant if the lemon wedge is too big. We dealt with the same women and smiled through it. Really they gave us quite a bit to laugh about most of the time.

"Here is the hard real truth about radiation. It is the loneliest frightening experiences of the hospital settings. Take it from me—I have a hospital chart that's as thick as a phone book. I'm still recuperating from my second craniotomy. The walk to radiation is itself a kind of mental torture. On your way to radiation there is hallway of rooms with people getting chemotherapy. The poor people at the end of these IV lines look like dying insects in various stages of their demise. I'm sorry if that sounds cruel but when you walk that hall on your way to radiation, it's a cruel lonely walk and it feels like a wicked world. The view into those rooms seemed like a glimpse into the future for me. It made me less than hopeful.

"On the bright side, the doctors, technicians, and nurses are wonderful. They are doing exactly what they should be doing. They are all sweet, caring people. Unfortunately, after they set you all up for radiation you are alone again."

Even someone as strong and positive as Susan W. feels lonely and frightened, and she experiences moments of "mental torture." Underlying it all, however, I hear the voice offering practical suggestions and realistic emotional support to other women—readers of this book—undergoing radiation, while she participates in research in order to help others. When I talk about "ordinary miracles," I have people like Susan W. in mind.

8

SUPPORT SYSTEMS: "AN EXTREMELY EMOTIONAL TIME FOR MY FAMILY AND FRIENDS"

"We have encountered four problems (in breast cancer patients), which may occur separately or in some combination and which we believe interfere with the return to emotional balance. The problems are difficulties in interpersonal relations, the revival of conflicts existing before diagnosis and treatment, repeated loss of functionality, and the continued intensification of emotional reactivity."
—Charlene A. Carter, Ph.D. and Ross E. Carter, Ph.D.,
Medical College of Wisconsin.

Two of the major themes of this book are, on the one hand, the hope, strength, and courage of "ordinary" women in pursuing the "miracle" of their recovery from cancer and, on the other hand, their reliance on a variety of support systems in accomplishing that miracle. We have seen evidence of that support in each of the chapters so far, but here I want to focus on support more specifically. I have found that the support comes from a variety of sources—family and friends, nurses and other health care professionals. These sources of support often complemented one another in sustaining the resilience of the breast cancer survivor. Another form of support, a "spiritual connection," will be the subject of the next chapter.

Let's hear first from Beatrice, who received practical and emotional support from her family: "Some thoughts on the doctor visits: my two daughters and my husband were always present. It's amazing how information is heard differently. How important it is to have more than one set of ears hearing what each doctor, nurse, or technician says. Not only does this help to give a clear picture of whatever is under discussion but one never feels alone."

She went on to elaborate on the emotional support that alleviated the feeling of being alone:

"So when friends and family offer to help in any way, it was easy to say, 'How nice—that would be much appreciated.' They became an addition to our lives, heartwarming and helpful. A visit with others always created a sense of wellness. The more open I was with others, the more they could feel a part of the recovery.

"Phone calls are tiring but also can become easy visits. I could decide how much I was able to do. People understand. Those who have supportive family and friends are most fortunate. The American Cancer Society, Gilda's Club, to name just two resources, are there for all who wish to use them. The support they give can be invaluable.

"Being an elderly woman with a spouse and grown children, all dedicated and thoughtful, made my experience easier than many. My responsibilities were nil and the excuse of tiredness allowed me to do what I wanted to do . . . without guilt.

"In December, my husband and I moved to Florida for the next 5 months. Our children and grandchildren visited us over the holidays. I felt whole, energetic, and normal, due to the loving period of family togetherness and/or being the third week before chemo."

True, we are not all blessed with "dedicated and thoughtful" children! But Beatrice knew how to ask for and accept their support, which I'm sure must have eased her experience—and her family's.

Another woman, Isamay, received similar family support: "Bob was as surprised as me with the news. He was immediately supportive (he is a colon cancer survivor, 10 years ago). Our son and daughter-in-law, too, were right there on the team. I had waited until I knew the results of the core biopsy before sharing all with my mom. At 83, and adjusting to a toe amputation, we felt she didn't need to worry about my test result. Once we knew, she was told, was surprised and, as a mom would be, supportive. She had experienced lumpectomies herself, although never had any radiation or chemotherapy."

Isamay saw her family as part of "the team," and as part of the team, she used her judgment in deciding when to tell her mother.

She continued to broaden her support network:

"My surgery was on a Monday morning. The following Thursday, we were to travel north (to Shanty Creek Resort) where my husband would preside over a statewide convention. I was responsible for the ladies' program (a luncheon on Saturday). Because I felt well and with the doctor's blessing, we kept our plans. On Friday, I rode in the golf cart and putted. Friday evening, I shared my surgical experience with a few close friends. At the ladies' luncheon, I shared all I knew about my surgery and what might be ahead, with all in attendance. We had not been 'public' to this point, because people are people and stories grow. But now was the time to tell. I told them each step, saying that further therapy would be determined in another week. I wanted these people to know what I knew and to hear the 'real' story from me. The outpouring of love and concern was incredible—not only from the women, but from the guys, too (unbeknownst to me, Bob was sharing our story at his meeting). It was maybe not so surprising that several gals told me they had gone through a breast cancer experience also. So my support team expanded to many friends and acquaintances throughout the state."

Isamay used the phrase "support team," and I love the way her husband enlisted others to be part of the team. I'm not certain, however, that all breast cancer survivors would want that to happen.

She went on to add, "Our pastor and church family certainly played a great role in my treatment and recovery process. It is wonderful to have the caring support of those around you."

We see similar positive support in the words of Georgina:

"As far as my family, they were great. My daughter is a registered nurse. She was very supportive and helpful. My husband was also supportive. He and I did many walks, gave donations, and did a lot of volunteering for various cancer groups.

"Some had had cancer in the past and were very supportive—sharing their experiences to alleviate my fears.

"My husband had just finished a long journey of health problems when I was diagnosed. He rose to the occasion and was fully able to pitch in and take care of every need."

And from Sharon:

"My boyfriend, Dick, accompanied me on that all-day educational experience. He was my rock and my crutch throughout the whole ordeal. My daughter lives 2 hours away and my son would have been uncomfortable caring for me and vice versa. Dick and I were totally impressed with the information gained and efficiency of the breast clinic. We felt secure to make a decision and entrust HFH with my treatment. We spent an entire day (8 A.M. to 6 P.M.) at the main hospital and met with all the specialists and had all the tests needed to make a plan of treatment. My children were both supportive and concerned."

I appreciate Sharon's use of the word "we."

Heidi elaborated on the kind of family support she received:

"My husband and I are acquainted with cancer (Tom had prostate cancer surgery in 1998, and I had breast cancer surgery in 1990). Both of us learned that a positive attitude helps us and our team of doctors, so that our reaction was to go forward and not to be afraid. Tom's and my parents are deceased, and we do not have any children. My immediate family (sister and brother and their families) live in Germany and the Netherlands, respectively. Our contact was by telephone. They reacted with sadness but were very encouraging. My sister experienced breast cancer in 1995, so she is familiar with the "ups and downs." My friends were supportive and distracted me from "doubtful" moments by keeping me busy.

"There are a few especially memorable experiences: first, my husband's patience and loving care to dress my wound and empty the drainage device three times a day (this lasted from February to May); the delicious homemade soups that some friends brought over; our tenth wedding anniversary we celebrated in late May at the Shaw Festival in Niagara-on-the-Lake at a charming

Victorian Bed & Breakfast home (with drainage device). And I was able to attend most of my choir rehearsals from February to May to participate in our Spring Concert performing two beautiful masses by J.S. Bach."

Sometimes, however, as in Lucille's case, the people around us let us down:

"Through it all, my husband was always very supportive (he is also a cancer survivor), but I chose to keep it to myself after seeing the reaction of many friends who didn't want to talk about it. Tennis friends were the worst. They seemed to be afraid it might rub off on them. But here I am, 71 years old in 2004 and still OK with 6-month checkups."

And Marianne discovered, "Family and neighbors were sympathetic and very kind. Some friends and coworkers suddenly became strangers." In a similar vein, Hardeep noted, "My friends were largely ignorant of how to react, either over- or underreacting." Toni reported that her family and friends treated her cancer "like a cold. Not as serious as I felt."

Roxanne said flatly: "My whole world caved in. To make matters worse, I live alone; all my family is in another state. Three friends of mine gave me a hand. One took me to the hospital, another picked me up, and the other one came every day that I was hospitalized for the last part of the treatment when it was intensified. I will limit myself to tell you that no one in my family could come."

Susan described a mixture of great support and a puzzling lack of support:

"My family was all shocked and concerned with the diagnosis but I think that, because I was so positive through it all, they felt relieved and were less frightened about the future. I am extremely fortunate to have two close cousins who are surgical and medical oncologists and I was able to get information, support, and reassurance from them. I will always be indebted to them—I couldn't have managed as well as I did, without their assistance. As for friends, I had some interesting reactions. Most people were extremely supportive, offering to bring meals and drive me to hospital appointments whenever I needed it, sending cards and phoning or emailing regularly. But there were a couple of friends that I never heard from during all the months of treatment. I think some people have a difficult time dealing with illness for different reasons."

I appreciate her forgiveness of her disappearing friends. It is not always easy to be a friend or family member of a breast cancer patient.

Sally Cole-Saul illustrated this difficulty with her account of her two instances of breast cancer:

"The first time no one could believe I had cancer because I was regarded by friends and family as a health nut; I had been and still was physically very fit and exercised regularly, participated in vigorous sports. I worked full-time and I was always in high gear on the job and at home, full of endless energy. My sister had passed away at 40 of breast cancer and everyone was aware of this. Because of this I often wondered how I would handle the big C, if I were confronted with it and had to tell my family and friends. Unfortunately when

I actually experienced this, the cancer and the issue of dealing with it, several times, the experience was not at all as expected.

"The first instance was an extremely emotional time for my family and friends, and there were many different reactions by others. My friends were the most helpful, but perhaps the most distressful aspect was the fact that the first time my mom minimized the entire experience (I felt that she regarded my health challenge and surgery as about as significant as a tonsillectomy). Her perspective was that I should just go and do what the doctor's recommended, have the surgery and whatever else, and then get back to life as normal (an 'ignore it and it will go away' kind of attitude or approach).

"The second time all she could say was how sorry she was, but I found no comfort or solace in this minimal communication from her. I had married after the first cancer, and during the second occurrence my husband was my biggest supporter, advocate, and source of comfort. He helped me research to find the best doctors and to evaluate the best procedures and to feel good about every decision that we made. Of most importance is probably that we both felt that we had done all we possibly could in the way of research and analysis and then made informed choices.

"During the second cancer, many of my friends did not know what to say, possibly because they did not understand the disease or were in denial or just plain at a loss for words in emotional times. It is one thing to hear about breast cancer, but unless you have been diagnosed with it, it is hard to relate or understand what goes on in the victim's mind and how to comfort someone facing this kind of life crisis."

Sally Cole-Saul generously moved to an understanding of the difficulty of those whose support is disappointing. She went on to note "the importance of support from family and friends—true support from sincere people who simply let you know that they care, that they are there for you, and that they will add their prayers and positive feelings to those of others for you."

One way to deal with missing or inappropriate efforts at support is through participating with a group, as Georgina described:

"I went to Gilda's Club every week to discuss all aspects of breast cancer . . . The people at Gilda's were very helpful to me—it was a God-send . . . Gilda's Club in Royal Oak was great. Everyone there was wonderful. The support of the people helped me get through a very frightening time of life."

Gilda's Club, a well-organized, community-supported cancer support organization, or organizations like it, can be found in most cities.

Sometimes, unfortunately, the spouse is the sole source of emotional support, as Judith described:

"I am lucky to have a very supportive husband as my doctor did nothing to help me with the shock of the diagnosis or what I was going through. My husband is always by my side and he is a great support. He had a heart transplant at Henry Ford in 1998 and so we have been through a lot together with his heart disease over 12 years. We pray and then face everything with a positive attitude, learn all we can about the situation, and take it one day at a time; which we did and got the best care at the best facility."

Georgina went on to note the difficulty in enlisting other family members who are themselves in need of support: "My Mom was very upset when I told her as my father died of cancer in 1998 and you always think of death when you hear the word. Our daughters were upset especially the youngest, who was 23 at the time."

But even those who are shocked and sickened can rally to offer support, as was the case with Becky: "Family and friends were shocked and sickened by my diagnosis. My soul mate Roy was scared for the both of us . . . Thank you, Roy, Gail, Vickie, and Mary for waiting 12 hours at the hospital for me to wake up."

Again and again we see ways that families offer support. Linda P. described her relationship with her family:

"My next task was to sit down with my four sons and explain it all to them— a job I wasn't looking forward to but, nonetheless, one that had to be done. Turns out it wasn't as bad as I expected since I have such a warm, loving family. They were very understanding and supportive and to this day they run and walk to raise money for cancer research and continue to pray for me and with their mom.

"My surgery was in September and in October I went to Las Vegas with my sister. I got a royal flush on a video poker machine (winning about $1,000). She and I split it for a happy holiday. She was my support along with my daughter during the whole ordeal."

Women like D'Anna, the "Brownie mom" we met earlier, often involved their younger children in a system of mutual support:

"I had decided very early on that this wasn't going to be a death sentence, but if it turned out that way, then I wanted to spend time with the girls. My older daughter was in second grade at the time and knew what the possibilities were. She was pretty freaked out about the situation and wanted to stay close by. But the other one was too young (in kindergarten) to understand much, other than the fact that she couldn't cuddle on my right side like we had been. It was a good excuse to have them go to sleep in their own beds instead of our bed. I just told them that I couldn't carry them back to their beds when it was time for me to go to bed! Both of them liked having me home when they got home from school. I told them over and over that we were doing everything possible so mommy would be around for a long time. I took them to see where I got chemo, and then later, they came with me: to see the radiation setup."

Husbands were often an integral part of the recovery team. Jennie described her relationship:

"I had a good nurse (my husband) who took care of the drainage and all my needs. Each time before surgery I tell my family, husband and two sons, that I love them all and God will watch over the operation and whatever happens is not in our hands. Then faith and prayers are powerful, and having a positive attitude is a must. My husband of 49 1/2 years has been my best support, nurse, housemaid, with a lot of love, care, and patience."

And in the following passage, Susan W.'s husband gets only a minor mention, but (as a husband!) I sense that he is an important part of her recovery experience:

"My husband and I had always planned to go to Hawaii for our twenty-fifth wedding anniversary. This just so happened to fall in that same year. We did not let my breast cancer stop us. Instead, we made our travel plans to coincide with the end of my chemo treatments. This was great because it was like the rainbow after the storm. It gave me something to look forward to.

"This was our second trip to Kauai. It is a beautiful island. The shrubs around the Sheraton Kauai Hotel bloom big red flowers and every lobby hallway and restaurant have big fresh sprays of exotic flowers. There is even a small fresh flower on every plate at every meal. These trips are business and pleasure. My husband gets sent through business and it is my pleasure to accompany him. The sound of the ocean waves pounding the shore lull you to sleep at night. These trips are always a welcome relief in the winter but never quite so much as this particular winter. I was a bit uncomfortable, but if you have to recuperate, Hawaii is my suggestion."

Sometimes husbands are not so successful in providing support, as we hear in the emotion in Beverly's concluding words: "Drs. G. and U. along with the nurses and technicians were a great support through this trying time. My three children, their spouses, and grandchildren were a great support; but I sensed my husband drawing away."

The complex kind of support that family and friends can provide is most evident in Jennie's story. Note how they wove in and out of the events and decisions:

"I always had my regular mammograms. I had one 3 months prior to my husband finding the lump on my left breast. I went to see my gynecologist who wanted me to have another mammogram done. When I went down to set up an appointment for this the receptionist making the appointments informed me she could not fit me in for a couple of weeks. One of the mammogram technicians happened to walk out and heard my pleas, 'I could not wait that long.' She immediately said she had time right then to perform the mammogram (an Angel sent from God). Before I even received the results back from that mammogram my sister, who had just recently finished her treatment from breast cancer, urged me to see her breast surgeon. Dr. V. is just a wonderful caring person. I had a needle biopsy done that same day. I believe that was on a Thursday and I had to wait until Monday for the test results. I am the type of person that handles things by myself, meaning, my husband never felt it necessary to go to a doctor's visit with me. That Monday he insisted on coming with me even though we both knew this was going to be nothing. My sister also magically just showed up that Monday. I believe God put it in their hearts that I would need them both. When Dr. V. walked in the room, he did not make eye contact with me. I knew at that moment that I had breast cancer. I do not really remember what his words were as I was crying and very upset. That day is just a blur! I will always remember the date, September 14, 1998, as it was my daughter's eighteenth birthday. She was away at college and I had to call her and give her the bad news. That was a very painful thing to do. That being said, in a couple of days we were back in to see Dr. V. about my options. The two options were a lumpectomy and a modified radical mastectomy. I opted for the mastectomy because that was the only way I would have peace of mind that the entire tumor was gone. Losing my breast was really not an issue for me as I felt I was in a fight for my life. As far as the thought of my husband not finding me attractive anymore was also nonissue. We are and always will be true soul mates."

Many of the breast cancer survivors were retired at the time of their treatment, but some who were working described meaningful support from their coworkers. Linda N. said, "With the help and support of my wonderful co-workers, I was able to work during my treatment. I had my work day shortened a couple of hours each day so I could have my radiation treatment in the morning." And D'Anna said:

"I went back to work the beginning of February and worked part-time during all my treatments. Because of a new policy at the hospital, I was allowed to work part-time while on disability. It was a financial hardship for us, but I was on half-time during chemo and three-quarter time during radiation. It was great to come and go as I wished, and my boss and the Division Head were very supportive. My boss said he would rather have me working part-time than not at all."

It is clear to me that the support being felt here is more than just practical. The women see an acknowledgment of their disease and of their value as human beings.

While the support of family and friends was profoundly valuable, the responses to our questionnaire revealed that doctors and nurses provided an equally important kind of emotional support in addition to the strictly medical work they performed. Listen to these voices, which I present without commentary.

From Roxanne: "My most memorable moments were with the nurses. They worked so hard and they were so sweet. When I showed up for the first time to receive my first chemotherapy, I sat quietly and patiently waiting for one nurse to come and begin the therapy. As I waited, I watched all of them. I chose two nurses. They were from the Philippines. I had another talk to God while I waited. Oh yes! I talk to Him all the time. 'I want Gloria,' I thought in my mind. It was important for me to have whom I chose. She came straight to me and she continued to be the nurse that assisted me. I made her laugh and she was just as sweet as she could be. I felt her spirit, full of kindness and love. This was very important to me, *very*. I knew God was listening and was doing little things for me to make me comfortable and ease the discomfort of my ordeal."

From Marianne: "Two technicians from Royal Oak HFH location took me to my empty office and prayed for me holding hands. I am not Christian and they are. It still gives me goose bumps remembering it."

From Beatrice: "I chose Dr. N. to be the surgeon. He is soft spoken, clear in his thoughts and speech, has great eye contact and is highly experienced. A recognition of the spiritual added to this sense of sureness." She continued: "The many tests that were given prior to the surgery made sure the heart was strong, the chest x-ray clear, and scans showing no other sign of cancer. The results were sent to me by my family practitioner, Dr. P. The report pleased her as noted by the happy faces she drew on this official document. Those happy faces pleased me too! Little things mean a lot. Full scale scans of the upper and lower intestines showed me to be healthy."

From Becky: "I did a lot of research and through good friends found Dr. N. and Henry Ford Hospital, which was a comfort, a godsend, and my second opinion. Did I mention Wanda? Wanda was the angel dressed as a nurse in charge of setting up my consultation with all the doctors. She treated me like we were best friends. I had nothing but good feelings right from the start, which carried me through the rest."

From Linda P.: "My doctor was wonderful through this ordeal—from beginning to the present. I know I can talk to him anytime and he will give me his time and words of wisdom." And from Lucille: "Then along came my angel, Sue, from Dr. D.'s office, who said, 'You don't have to look like that, go for reconstruction.' It didn't take long for me to make up my mind. For someone who lives in a bathing suit in Florida all winter and played tennis, it was the only way to go."

From Susan W.: "I would like to thank Dr. N., Dr. G., the nurses, and technicians at Henry Ford in West Bloomfield. Thank you for being who you are and your sense of humor and for never making me feel self-conscious. Thank you for making me a part of your brilliant study. I have recommended you highly. I would also like to thank other Michigan Organizations for coming to Hudson's in the late 1990s to show slides and more important, show us hands on what to look for in your breast. Most of us knew about it and did self-examination, but they had teaching tools that were of monumental help. I knew exactly what I had found that night, because it felt just like what they gave me to feel. I would love to be in a program that provided a service such as this. If I am needed, please let me know. I would love to help someone else."

From Linda N.: "My journey began with an amazing person, Dr. S. She was, at that time, a mammography radiologist for the Henry Ford System. She literally took me by the hand and walked me through every procedure prior to my surgery. Dr. S. was the one who recommended Dr. N. to do my surgery."

From Georgina: "Most memorable was meeting a wonderful doctor named Dr. A. He answered all my questions about breast cancer."

"I shopped around to find an oncologist that made me feel comfortable. I found Dr. A. at Fairlane Clinic. Another radiation patient told me about him—I think it's very important to compare notes with other cancer patients because then you can pick the best treatment plan for yourself."

From Margaret: "Most memorable were the comfort (both physical and spiritual) and friendship of the nurses, etc., in the hospital." And from Sonja: "Dr. N. asked if I would be interested in being a participant in a clinical trial with a new procedure called sentinel 'first' node biopsy. He explained the procedure to me and I said OK. After talking with him, I felt a peace within and a feeling that everything was going to be all right. My most memorable experience was the compassion and kindness of the medical staff. I am a retired nurse, and I know the importance of being a kind and caring person to your patients. I wish to thank all my doctors, nurses, and the staff in the radiation department for taking good care of me."

From Alyce: "The care and love shown by Henry Ford is unbelievable. The nurses, the doctors, and aides all have such a calmness that is ever so soothing." And from Toni: "Dr. N.'s bedside manner and reassurance. "

From Jennie: "I thank each and all of my special doctors who have helped me through each ordeal. I do see Dr. B, Oncology, Dr. G., who has been very thorough with my health. Thank you Dr. N. for the lymph node test. Also Dr. J.G. and his special nurse who explained everything to me and my husband. All my family gave me support, and mammograms are very important. We take them every year."

Eve took special pains to thank her doctors by name and title. Her situation was especially difficult, moving first to Detroit from another country and then to another city for her continued treatment:

"I would like to say a few words about the feeling of arriving in a new city that actually I was visiting a lot of times but I did not have a doctor to talk to about my problems. Family doctors are not personal doctors. I moved to Cleveland in May 2002 because I got my citizenship in November 2001. To leave Detroit with my good treatment was not easy. I was looking for good doctors that could help me. I was lucky that a friend of mine introduced me to her primary doctor, Dr. S. He is not just a very good doctor but also a wonderful human being. So I had a good beginning. My daughter working in the University Hospital talked to Dr. L., breast/surgeon/oncologist, and I was lucky that she did my left breast lumpectomy. She is a very serious and wonderful doctor. Also with my daughter's help I was accepted by Dr. K., hematologist/oncologist, and she recommended me to go through the bone scan, CT scan, blood test, x-ray before she decided that I must take Arimidex every day one tablet if I do not want to get more lumps in my breast. This is a better medicine for me because it does not attack the arteries. I hope I will be able to take it as long as I will need it. I have been taking this medicine since 2/6/2004. I got my radiation therapy from Dr. L., Director, Radiation/Oncology breast service. She is also a very serious and good doctor and I feel lucky to be in hood hands. I began my treatment on 3/1/04 and I need 31 treatments. I hope that everything will be OK but nobody can predict the future. So far so good, thank God. Today is 4/12/04 and I finished the radiation therapy. Thank God everything is OK with me: I take my Arimidex and I feel healthy, and I am full of hope that this medicine is better for me. In the future I will follow my checkup mammograms, and help myself with good healthy diet and exercises. I will do everything that is in my hand to be able to enjoy life because I have a passion for life. The alternative is much worse and we all will find out sooner or later what is this other world."

Eve's passion for life is another underlying theme expressed in the stories of all these cancer survivors.

Breast cancer survivors are typically very resourceful in locating needed support systems. Sally Cole-Saul, whose difficulties in garnering support from family and friends we saw earlier in this chapter, also noted:

"In 1993 my doctor suggested I join a support group, which I did. This was somewhat helpful in that it made me realize that many others were similarly afflicted and that there were many people with a worse prognosis than mine, and much more to deal with—some had small children, some had not yet had children and wanted to, etc.

"In 1998, my oncologist reviewed the mammogram and simply advised us to set up a surgery immediately and see what we learned. This approach exacerbated an already stressful state for me. My husband and I sought a second opinion from the University of Michigan Hospital (outside our health care plan) where I had relatives. The U of M staff suggested we also consider Henry Ford Hospital and the Josephine Ford Cancer Center Breast Cancer Clinic.

"At the Josephine Ford Cancer Center Breast Cancer Clinic my experience was very key in getting over the emotional aspects of this second incidence of cancer. Dr. N., the Department Director and the clinic staff treated us in a calm and professional manner and responded to our endless and sometimes redundant questions without any indications of impatience or exasperation on their part. Because we sought the knowledge to reach the best decisions, we were pleased that they did not just give us advice (although likely they would have if we had wanted them to), but instead we felt very comfortable that we received from them what we needed to feel good about making the right decisions. I believe that what helped me the most in dealing with the fact was that we were confident up front in the competency of the doctors and staff and that we felt comfortable with our decisions. It was not just about what we learned but about how we learned it and the environment in which we learned it."

Resourcefulness is the key in these ordinary miracles. The breast cancer survivors whose stories we tell here were not superhuman, but they were able to find ways to draw upon family, friends, and coworkers in order to magnify their strength. In the next chapter, we will see how many survivors also drew upon a spiritual connection to help them in their struggles.

9

THE SPIRITUAL CONNECTION: "MAKE ME FEEL LIKE A WHOLE PERSON"

The spiritual connection reported by people who responded to the questionnaire was a form of support that took a number of forms—some direct and some indirect.

Bettie felt the connection in a simple and direct way: "People all over the United States and Hawaii were praying for me." Alyce described what appeared to be direct benefits of her spiritual connection: "The surgery was outpatient and little or no problem. My family was completely supportive, but concerned. I do have deep faith in God and I placed my problem in God's hands ... My God helped me. I had no pain."

Jackie described benefits of similar faith: "I want to start out by thanking the Lord Jesus Christ for guiding me through my battle with breast cancer. He blessed me with a loving husband and a family that was always there for me."

Margaret said, "St. Jude was and still is my main support and spiritual connection." And Sally Cole-Saul, whose resourcefulness we noted earlier, said, "I prayed every night and I still do for God to watch over me and my family and friends. I felt that the many prayers from my family and friends and from others that I did not personally know had a positive effect on my surgery and my recovery. While I do not attend church regularly, I do have a strong belief and I do know that prayer really does work!" She went on to emphasize "the power of prayer and belief in God and oneself."

Others, such as Hardeep, found their spiritual support outside of the Christian religion: "My spiritual connection was through my Gurdwara (Sikh temple), through prayer, meditation, and Reiki."

The most deeply and fully expressed sense of spiritual support is this from Clara, who we have met before:

"Until I needed the biopsy I was petrified when they gave me the diagnosis. I am a born-again Christian. I prayed and asked the Lord to remove this cup (of God's spirit) from me. Nevertheless, not my will, but thine be done.

"The dermatologist said she would have the surgeon and all his staff meet me, so I would be acquainted and not alarmed. That was good. They were all wonderful, so reassuring. But I still wasn't sure I should go through the operation. They said I could cancel if I wanted to.

"I told my daughter. She said, 'Mom, you've got to.' I was sort of in a state of shock and disbelief, and I hoped it would go away and be healed. God had healed me of so many things before where I didn't need an operation. But I didn't see it healing, so I relented and went to the surgeon, Dr. N.

"I thank the Lord, and HFH and the doctors and staff *for healing* and such good care and getting the cancer out."

Clara goes on to elaborate on her spiritual connection:

"I renounced Satan, repented and asked Jesus to wash me with His Blood, forgive, love, and teach me the will and way. I was baptized in the Father-Son-Holy Ghost, and was given the Holy Spirit to live in me: the seal upon my heart that I belong to God through Jesus Christ. I attend the Emmanuel Lutheran Church in Dearborn. I am so thankful Jesus came from Heaven to be born in a Virgin (the Seed of God in the Virgin Mary). Jesus Christ became the (God–Man) fully God–fully Man, so He could die as a man for our sins and pay our sin debt, and rise from death as God, giving us eternal life. He buried our sins and took back the keys Satan stole from Adam and Eve, and preached in hell and rose, was seen by a few, went to the father, was glorified, came back, was seen of many, had communion with His disciples, and was lifted up into heaven as they watched Him go, where He is now—seated at the father's right hand, our Advocate, High Priest, Lord, Savior. He will return in the clouds to call all who Received Him to come up with Him. So shall we ever be with the Lord (see 1 Thessalonians 4:13–18). We must confess our sins (1 Jn 1:9) go and sin no more deliberately, knowingly. We must also confess in sincere faith Jesus is God come in the flesh to save us, that He is the Lord and alive (see Romans 10:4,10). He didn't say all would be fair weather, but trials, troubles, temptations, burdens, cares, etc. But we could cast all our cares upon Him, for He cares for us: I do and read God's Word (Genesis through Revelations) a portion every day.

"I did have fear at first, not of dying. I didn't want to be an invalid. But then I listened to the Lord's Word: 'I will be with you.' So even if I died, I would be with Him. And all at Henry Ford Hospital were so reassuring, kind, gentle, and positive. Satan was having a field day, but Jesus won the victory! (See Col. 2:9—Hallelujah, Hallelujah, Hallelujah!)"

Others, such as Heidi, found their spiritual connection in a less direct way:

"My husband and I have been active members of the Fort Street Presbyterian Church in downtown Detroit for the last 12 years. I have a postwar Christian upbringing in the Reformed Church in my hometown in northern Germany. FSPC has a liberal and diversified congregation with many outreach programs to the community. My favorite program is the Fort Street Chorale. I love to sing and enjoy sacred music. The Chorale performs for the public in May and December. Our May concerts consist of requiems, masses, oratorios, and Handel's *Messiah* is our December program (for the last 25 years, and it has been a sellout every year). To make music is a wonderful way to feel at ease, feel comforted, and have peace of mind. The Chorale is more than making music together; joy and sorrow are shared by all members."

At the end of her response to the questionnaire, she added this note:

"I would like to add another chapter [to this book]. Most of the support comes through family, friends, spiritual connections, or other groups. My experience is self-help. Listening to music (in my case it's mainly classical), as I mentioned before I sing in a choir (I am not a trained singer, but my heart is in it), reading, walking, taking a low-impact aerobics class, cooking a healthy meal for myself or a loved one, attending live concerts and theater performances; these are positive distractions from any concerns and worries and make me feel like a whole person."

Music and aerobics can certainly work in a spiritual way for some people. Again, the breast cancer survivors were amazingly resourceful in finding what works for them. Marianne's response to our question about spiritual connection underscores that point:

"I have no formal spiritual connections. I am spiritual and tried a number of alternative medications following my treatments and I still do. Gilda's Club was very helpful."

I'm impressed with the variety of ways these women found to locate and create their support systems. There is no single answer. Some turned to family and friends. Others found support in the health care professionals and organizations such as Gilda's Club. Many found support through organized religion, while others saw support in the spiritual aspects of music and theater. Some placed a great deal of trust in God and in doctors, while others emphasized self-reliance—God was strengthening them and guiding their doctors, and the patients themselves were active members of the team that was supporting them.

One person, Rosalba Primavera Pacella, described in detail a kind of spiritual support that she calls "The Miracles of Angels on Earth." You will see how she presents an integrated blend of family and spiritual support:

November 30, 1995 is a day that I will never forget. It was the beginning of a miracle that I call "angels on earth."

The year 1989 was the beginning of my brother Nick's battle against breast cancer. He was only 37 years old. He was happily married with a loving wife and two beautiful children whom he adored. One day he discovered a lump in his breast and made an appointment with his family doctor to get it checked. After being examined, Nick was referred to a well-known surgeon for evaluation; the doctor's opinion was: it is nothing to worry about. He asked, "What are the chances of a man having breast cancer?"

A year or so went by and Nick was still worried about the lump that grew in his breast. He had made several trips to the surgeon's office, but nothing was done about the lump.

A date was set for Nick to have surgery, not because of the lump, but because of a hernia that needed immediate attention. Nick took this opportunity to request that the lump on his breast be removed because he was not comfortable with its being there, and the surgeon agreed to remove it. Everyone in our family was concerned about his surgery (because there is always a risk any time an individual has an operation). However, we were confident that everything would be fine. No one had prepared us for what was about to happen: our world crashing down on us, most of all on Nick and his wife and children. The doctor coming out of surgery in shock gave my sister-in-law the bad news: "It is breast cancer."

Cancer is a word that no one ever wants to hear. There was no history of cancer in our family. How could this be? Was this a mistake? What were they going to do next? Could they save him? Was I going to lose my big brother? How was I going to tell my parents, who were thousands of miles away from us and did not have a clue about any of this? I had so many questions and no answers. All I could do was pray, and ask God for a miracle, the miracle of life.

The day after all of this madness, a second surgery was preformed on Nick to remove any cancer that was left behind. Many lymph nodes were removed and sent out to be checked by a lab. At that time we did not have sentinel lymph node biopsy to determine which lymph nodes were cancerous. When the results came back a few were positive, and Nick needed several treatments of chemo.

Time went on and Nick seemed to be doing better. He went back to work but was always worried that the cancer would return.

In November 1995, his fear became a reality. He was rushed to the hospital by ambulance after passing out at work. A CAT scan was done of his brain. After a long waiting period the doctor walked into his room and said, "You have a brain tumor, and I am pretty sure that it has metastasized from your breast." No one could comfort Nick. He was crying hysterically and could not say a word.

A few days later surgery was performed, and a tumor, the size of a golf ball, was removed from his brain. He was left partially paralyzed from the surgery. He was told, "You are going to need radiation and a lot of aggressive therapy, you won't be able to drive anymore, and you won't be able to work."

Nick was devastated. All he knew was work; he had been working since he was 12 years old. As time went by he learned to accept it, he did not feel sorry for himself, and he did not want pity from anyone. He always looked at people that had it worse than him. He was thankful to be alive and to see his children grow up.

Five years went by and the cancer returned, this time in his spine. After two major surgeries and treatments I could tell the end was near. I tried to spend as much time with him as I could. He enjoyed talking about all his spiritual experiences that he had throughout these years and told me that he was not afraid to die because he had seen heaven in a dream. He went on by telling me that the previous night angels came to visit him. I looked at him and thought that he was kidding me because he knew how much I believed in angels. "You should have been here," he said. "This room was full of angels. They were climbing on my bed and on the dresser. They were baby angels and they were all dressed in pink, only one of them was dressed in blue." I knew then that he was not kidding, that he really had seen a team of angels.

On November 30, 1995, the day after my brother's surgery, my mom and I went to the hospital to visit Nick. We walked into his room, and I could tell that he was in a lot of discomfort. His head was all bandaged up. Tears began rolling down my face. I felt helpless because my big brother, the one who was always there for me, was in great need, but there was nothing I could do for him to lessen his pain. How could this be? Why was this happening? Why Nick?

Nick looked at me and then looked at his wife. "Tell my sister not to look at me," he said. I did not want to see him upset, so I left the room. I sat by myself on a chair in the waiting area by the elevator, crying my eyes out and questioning God. Why Nick? I prayed to God to get him through this and to spare his life.

A young woman approached me. She was dressed in old-fashioned clothes as if she just stepped out of another century. She tried to start up a conversation with me, but I didn't pay much attention to her, so she left the waiting area. I was left there along with my questions and my anger. I wanted answers. Is there really a God? Why does he allow all this suffering? Why wasn't he helping Nick? What did Nick ever do that he deserved to suffer like that? He was a good person, always willing to help others. Why? God! In the meantime the woman that had approached me before returned.

She sat by me and introduced herself as Magdalene and asked, "Why are you crying?" I began to open up to her and told her how sick my brother was and how worried I was.

At this time she got up from her chair grabbed my hand and said to me, "Your brother has always been there for you, hasn't he?"

"Yes," I replied.

"Did you tell him that you have seen him at his worst and that you still love him?" I just looked at her with tears in my eyes. "Once in a while God shakes us up," she said, "because if everything goes our way we forget about Him."

She went on to say, "Jesus is my brother. Let's pray for your brother. I know you are in despair and you don't believe, but you must not lose your faith. Everything that happens, happens for a reason, and God knows what is best for us. When God calls upon your brother it is because that is what is best for him. He has a better place waiting for him; a place were there is no pain, no suffering, only peace."

The amazing thing is that when this woman was holding my hand and praying I felt something that cannot be described or explained, a sense of peace that I have never known. Her eyes and mine were locked together, her voice was soft and soothing. I wasn't aware of my breathing, my heartbeat, or anything around me. I felt safe, secure, and at peace.

I heard a voice that seemed to be coming from far away (when in fact it came from behind me). It was my mother checking up on me. "Rosalba, who is this woman?"

I answered, "She claims that Jesus is her brother!"

"Jesus is her brother?" my mother replied. "Maybe she is an angel," my mom said (in Italian). I looked at the lady who had comforted me in my time of need and translated what my mom had said.

She hugged me and said, "No, I am not an angel, but thank you, you helped me a lot."

"No," I replied, "you are the one who helped me. I was here all alone crying and you came to comfort me."

"We helped each other then. God spoke these words: 'When two or more gather together in my name and pray, I am in their midst.'"

My mother and I said goodbye to Magdalene and went back to Nick's room. We spent a few minutes with him, said our goodbyes, and went on our way. As we headed toward the hallway, there she was again, right across from Nick's room. (At the time I thought what a coincidence, but now I now that there are no coincidences in life, everything is already planned.) Standing there with another woman she introduced to us as her mother.

I have told this story to family members, friends, and acquaintances. Some of them believe just like me that she was a messenger of God who came to comfort me in my time of need. Others think that I felt something that wasn't really there. I have always believed in angels and feel that they are here for us when we need them. My experience was extraordinary, one that I wouldn't trade for anything.

I came to the conclusion that some things cannot be explained and we should not question why. Although God is in control, we do have a choice in the way we react. We all make mistakes, after all we are only human, but what is important is that we learn from them. We all have lessons to learn and we are on this earth to do God's work. That alone is a miracle.

On July 29, 2003, my loving brother lost his battle against breast cancer. What a fighter he was. What an inspiration he was to me and to so many people. His faith in God and his will to live were amazing. He was a believer of what our eyes could not see. He had faith, not fear. He fought the cancer with everything he had till the end. He loved his family so much, and he was convinced that he was going to beat it. However, his journey on earth was over, and God called him home. Saying goodbye to my brother was the hardest thing I ever had to do. But he left us with many beautiful memories, and left behind a legacy: *a team of angels*: www.teamangelsfoundation.org.

As he took his last breath he took a piece of my heart with him. I said, "Goodbye, Nick!" Kissed him on his forehead and told him that I loved him and that I would see him in my dreams. From the corner of my eye I saw a bright light. It reminded me of the bright light that he kept on seeing weeks before he passed. I knew then that he was in the arms of an angel and on his way home to be with God.

Whatever one's feelings may be about angels, I could not help but be moved by this story because of the depth of support that the writer describes. She was there for her brother, she experienced her own spiritual connection, and then she converted her grief into a drive "to do God's work," giving to others the miraculous support that she personally experienced. While this story breaks from the pattern of this book in that the story is not told by a breast cancer survivor, the theme of human strength and resourcefulness in the face of the terrible fact of cancer is one that we have seen again and again.

10

CASE STUDY—WENDY GOLDBERG: "I AM HERE"

HOW MY BREAST CANCER WAS DISCOVERED

It's remarkable, isn't it? In most contexts, references to private body parts and personal ailments are taboo. In the context of a serious diagnosis, however, that taboo is broken—in the doctor's office to be sure, but also among one's family, friends, and even in wider social circles that include colleagues and members of the community. For years, the knowledge that I had dense breast tissue was a private piece of data, rarely thought about and only referenced during my yearly mammograms when the good news of benign (noncancerous) findings were always accompanied by the caveat: "Extremely dense breast tissue could obscure a lesion on mammography." Good news, but don't count on it, was the way this message came across to me. I had always had dense tissue, and with three physicians (internist, gynecologist, and a surgeon) doing yearly examinations, plus my own breast self-examinations (BSEs), and with no family history of breast cancer, I just assumed everything was fine. There were the occasional palpable, suspicious lumps, but all of those biopsies proved to be negative (thank goodness).

A few years ago I noticed articles about the benefits of ultrasound as an adjunctive screening tool for individuals with dense breast tissue in some of my nurse practitioner journals. This information floated around in the back of my head until 2001 when my physicians, finding the usual collection of lumps and bumps, recommended a mammogram and an ultrasound. I asked the radiologist to do a bilateral ultrasound, and she complied. However, I discovered with hindsight a year later that it was a rather cursory examination— pleasant, polite, quick, and superficial; perhaps because the "official word" was that ultrasound wasn't yet an effective screening tool since it produced too many false positive results. I received the good news, and didn't look back; that is, until the following year.

The summer of 2002, my three "routine checkups" happened to be within weeks of each other. Curiously, my internist, gynecologist, and surgeon all felt breast lumps that concerned them, but none of these areas overlapped. To make matters more complicated, I felt a fourth area that the physicians hadn't identified. This time I knew I was going to insist on a bilateral ultrasound as a follow-up to the mammogram. On my way to the mammogram, I remember thinking, "This is so unscientific. Women with dense tissue like my own go through a process (mammography) that doesn't give them very useful information." If small tumors are often missed, I didn't want to just "go through the motions" of a screening process. I wanted the same chance as other women (with less dense tissue) to detect small tumors. Who needed meaningless reassurance? I wanted something I could count on better than mammogram alone, and ultrasound seemed to offer that advantage.

When the ultrasound technician asked me to point to the "area of concern," I laughed a little and said, "Sadly there are at least five different areas, and they are in both breasts, so I'd like you to do a bilateral ultrasound." The tech insisted that I identify one chief concern, to which I replied that the patient should not have to discriminate between her three physicians' findings and her own self-examinations as if this were a lottery. The only logical approach under these circumstances is to do a whole breast examination. Understandably, the tech had to follow her protocol, so I picked one of the lumps, and the tech proceeded to spend the next 20 minutes imaging, measuring, and recording information about this one small bit of tissue. She did her job. My only objection was that even after I identified myself as a Nurse Practitioner, she insisted on reminding me of the wisdom of the protocol. I promised to be cooperative, but had to insist that the tech refrain from rationalizing a set of general rules that did not fit my circumstance.

When the radiologist entered the room, a physician I had never met before very professionally presented the rationale for the "company line," which supported the use of targeted ultrasound (imaging suspicious lumps), but not whole breast ultrasound. I argued the merits of my request as they applied to my medical history, and we seesawed back and forth for a while locked in heated, but respectful dialogue. Remember, I was lying on a narrow examining table, covered with only a thin sheet. This is not exactly a position of authority. Maintaining my resolve instead of dissolving into the "obedient patient" was a bit of a struggle. Was I insane to persist? The urge to jump off the table was trumped by the conviction that the real insanity would be repeating an ineffectual practice just because it was currently the "standard of care."

The kind radiologist reminded me that with the high rate of false positives in screening ultrasounds I might be exposed to "needless worry." My immediate retort, "I'm a mature woman. I can handle worry. What I don't want to handle is a delayed diagnosis." Silence. And then the radiologist replied with quiet conviction, "You're right. That's why I do one every year on my wife." I shot back immediately, "Well today, you're going to do one on me." Logic prevailed.

Please keep in mind that I did not suspect I had cancer. The point is that if screening tests are a good idea, then people with dense breast tissue need an effective test just like everyone else. In contrast to the previous year's examination, the radiologist took his time, all the while pointing out areas of healthy tissue. He was so reassuring that during a pause in his verbal summation, I began to sit up, assuming the test was complete. "Well, there *is* one area of concern," he said as I sank back onto the table. "This hypoechoic area on the lower portion of your right breast needs a biopsy."

"Then get me one!" I practically commanded. After nearly falling to pieces while arguing my case for the ultrasound, I was determined now to maintain my composure. If a biopsy was needed, that's what I wanted—instantly, if possible. I believed it would turn out happily ever after like all the others—benign, benign, benign. By the way, this "area of concern" wasn't any of the previously identified suspicious lumps that my internist, gynecologist, surgeon, or I had been focusing on. The mammogram taken that day was read as normal and the tech had imaged healthy tissue, thus my cancerous lesion would not have been discovered if it were not for the use of ultrasound technology in the hands of the thorough radiologist.

In order to get the recommended biopsy, I was told to schedule an appointment in the breast clinic so that I could meet with a nurse and my surgeon. I've known Dr. N. for many years and regard him as a friend, dear colleague, and excellent physician. Nonetheless, I didn't want to engage in all this falderal. I just wanted the biopsy. If it turned out to be cancer, I reasoned, then I'd meet with the full cast of characters. No, I was told, *this* was the way it had to be done. To this day, I thank (nurse) Milica Kay for insisting that I accept this comprehensive approach to the diagnostic work-up. One of the best things about that difficult time was meeting Milica and knowing that I had at least two competent and supportive allies in the surgical department. The core needle biopsy (six show-stopping 1-second stings) was performed by the same radiologist who did the ultrasound. I trusted him to be thorough.

How I Felt When I Was Given the Diagnosis

I work as a Psychiatric Nurse Practitioner in the same health care system where I receive most of my health care. So, every day I checked the computer for the pathology report to see what the biopsy showed. This may be a bit irregular, but it is certainly my preferred way of doing things. For two days straight, I checked (sometimes hourly) for the report, and found nothing. On the third day, I checked the record 5 minutes before calling in my last outpatient of the day, and there it was: Infiltrating ductal carcinoma. I opened and closed the report half a dozen times, as if I might eventually hit upon a more favorable result. With my heart pounding, I called Milica who proceeded to track down Dr. N., and then I called my husband. "Not good," was all I could muster.

"I'll be right over." (Hal's office is only 15 minutes from the hospital.)

I answered Dr. Nathanson's page. "Where are you?" he queried.

"In my office," I whimpered.

"I'm coming over."

"Not until I see one more patient," I replied, setting our first postdiagnosis face-to-face meeting for about 4:00 P.M. that Friday afternoon.

Two seconds later I tried to suppress an escalating cascade of emotions while I escorted my patient from the waiting room to my office. Following the session (not my finest hour as a therapist, to be sure), I notified my secretaries and my supervising psychiatrist of my diagnosis. All offered to relieve me of any remaining duties for the day, but for a few minutes I clung to the belief that I could remain composed enough to do my job. After all, cancer didn't have to overtake my identity as a nurse and a mature adult. I found out quickly that composure was neither possible nor even reasonable at that moment. The more I spoke with my colleagues, the more the floodgates opened. People are so used to seeing me take charge in a crisis that I think they found it difficult at first to know how to respond. Normally, I'm the warm, comforting source for patients, families, and many colleagues. At a time when I just wanted to melt into someone's arms, the first few people I spoke with were kind, but a little distant. I present such a controlled demeanor most of the time, I think I was a little hard to read even with salt water pouring down my cheeks. Mark Ketterer, a psychologist I work with, did leave a little note in my office mailbox that afternoon saying simply, "Thinking about you." That helped.

What My Doctor Did to Help Me over the Initial Shock

When Dr. N. arrived, he immediately wrapped his arms around me in a secure, supportive gesture. It might be hard to imagine that there is such a thing as a professional hug, but trust me, there is. Just as Dr. N. sat down, my husband arrived, tearful and in shock. I sat in my office chair (after offering it first to Dr. N.), and the two men sat where my patients usually perch, Dr. N. in a chair, and my husband on the little couch. Most of the conversation is a blur. I do remember that Dr. N. outlined a plan of action that allowed us to proceed at my preferred rapid pace. He was going on vacation soon, so he wanted to schedule the surgery for the very next week. Dr. N. worked with a fellow staff member (Nurse Coordinator, Wanda Szymanski, R.N.) over the weekend to schedule all the necessary pre-op appointments and tests. I do remember trying to explain my views on quality of life and end of life care in the remote chance that something would go wrong during the surgery. Dismissive of the idea, but not of me, Dr. N. wasn't having any part of this catastrophic thinking.

Dr. N.'s help came in many forms that momentous day, and has continued throughout my illness and recovery. There are so many standout moments in our doctor–patient relationship. Some of the most memorable acts that Friday afternoon included: (1) offering to meet in my office, sparing me the trauma of a long walk to his office (in another building) where I'd invariably bump into people I knew along the way, (2) refraining from chastising me for looking up my own pathology report, (3) greeting me with a hug, (4) offering hopeful, clear, matter-of-fact explanations, (5) listening to my husband and me in an unhurried and receptive way, (6) being willing to get things rolling (appointments, testing, surgery) even though it meant working on the details through the weekend, and (7) accurately anticipating, and then voicing out loud what we would be facing that weekend as we shared this upsetting news with our family and large circle of friends.

Although this book is about Dr. N.'s work with cancer patients, I think he would be the first to point out that many physicians, indeed, many health care professionals, contribute to a patient's well being during immensely stressful times. I'd like to briefly mention a few of these individuals. Dr. B., an oncologist, friend, and colleague said something in the past that steadied my confidence during the first weeks of my breast cancer diagnosis. Years ago, when facing just the *possibility* of a cancer diagnosis after a breast biopsy, I said, "I can't do this," thinking how disruptive a diagnosis would be to my family and my work, and fearing that I could die.

"Yes you can," he firmly replied. Brilliant! I didn't feel admonished or negated. I actually felt reassured by his affirmation. I wouldn't have been comforted by, "It's probably nothing." (Often true, but a platitude nonetheless.) I wouldn't have been comforted by, "Why do you say that?" (I had a long list of ready, though incorrect, answers). I'm a fan of open-ended questions and empathic responses, but there's a time for plain directive statements, and this was it. "Yes you can," echoed in my head after the diagnosis, and helped me beat back overwhelming fear.

Dr. B. also telephoned soon after the diagnosis to inquire how I was doing. Once again, he put me at ease. I had considered asking him to be my oncologist, because his philosophy of caring and his approach to medicine compliment my own. However, I wasn't so sure if this was a good idea given our friendship and close collegial ties. I was in no emotional condition to initiate this sensitive conversation, and, as it turned out, I didn't have to. On the first phone call he said, "I just want you to know that I can be a friend when a friend is needed, and a doctor when a doctor is needed. Please don't feel any obligation to choose me for your physician. I can help you find good physicians. However, I do want you to know that should you wish, I would be happy to care for you."

What could be more reassuring? After my surgery, Dr. B. took it upon himself to contact the pathologist in the lab, and discovered, even before the report was issued, that my first surgery did not remove the entire tumor, and that I would need a second surgery. This quick action allowed me to return to the operating room 6 days later with Dr. N. If we had waited for the official pathology report, Dr. N. would have been out of town on vacation. Like Dr. N., Dr. B. spoke to me in a straightforward manner, and passed along relevant articles when questions arose about treatment options. He said the word "anxiety" out loud. He asked questions and actually waited for the answers.

My Nurse Practitioner friend, Cathy Baldy, and my Social Worker friend, JoAnne Ellis, took on the responsibility of notifying people at work, sparing me much emotional strain and allowing me to focus more on my family than my colleagues for the first month or so after the diagnosis. I knew Cathy and

JoAnne would know just what to say, how much, and to whom. I knew they would look after people's emotional needs as well as colleagues' reasonable requests for information.

Dr. D. was the oncologist assigned to the multidisciplinary breast cancer clinic on the morning of my appointment there, just 3 days after my diagnosis. Still in shock and having spent most of the weekend on the telephone crying with family and friends, I was not looking forward to seeing all these colleagues Monday morning as their new patient. In fact, I didn't look forward to the whole idea of sitting among other patients watching videos and being given "the drill" about an identity (cancer patient) I hadn't assumed yet. Let me tell you, one of the great benefits of this 3-hour clinic is its function as a rite of initiation into the patient role. The video, nurse's presentation, and meeting with physicians (surgeon, radiation oncologist, and oncologist) break through the shock and denial, transforming one from any old citizen to well cared for cancer patient. Entering this world is upsetting, but I left that day feeling steadied by the coordinated system of care, and the kind and able people delivering it. One standout moment was when shy, reserved Dr. D. greeted me with a spontaneous hug, exclaiming something like, "Oh, Wendy, I couldn't believe my eyes when I saw your name on the patient list." During a medical crisis facts are necessary, but so are warmth and empathy.

The above actions might seem so obvious as to be unworthy of mention. However, a small number of caregivers (unwittingly to be sure) offered meaningless, or worse, offensive platitudes. "Everything happens for a reason," is only reassuring if the patient believes it. Caregivers should not be the first to utter such a statement. It doesn't help when clinicians boldly try to identify the benefits of a crisis on the sufferer's behalf. To all those who told me, "Now you'll have a deeper understanding of your patients' viewpoints," I say, patients and staff have benefited from my imperfect counsel for many years. It is not necessary to risk one's life in order to achieve excellence. Furthermore, do we ask male obstetricians to become pregnant or psychiatrists to become psychotic, or heaven forbid, suicidal, in order to effectively minister to their patients? I will be the first to admit that I learned much about life and love and living from my illness, but I'm not happy that I became ill. Each time these other individuals told me how I would or should feel, how I would or should think, they were mistaken on all counts.

So, you can imagine how comforting it was when the Ambulatory Hematology/Oncology Supervisor, Deneen Ihlenfeldt, R.N., suggested that I take a tour of the Oncology Clinic through my new eyes as a cancer patient. I was very familiar with the physical plant. What Deneen was seeking was my input on the best way to receive care. There were several options, and she wanted me to be able to consider each one with the reassurance that she and her staff were totally at ease with whatever selection I made. Deneen knew I wouldn't want to trouble anyone, or make my case "special" in a prima donna kind of way. However, Deneen recognized that I needed not only excellent technical care but also the kind of privacy that all patients require to cope with the some-what unpredictable emotional and physical symptoms that usually accompany cancer treatment. Caring for a staff member, many of whose patients could be sitting in chairs right next to hers in the chemo room, presented a certain set of unique challenges. There are many "right" answers to these challenges. The cool thing is that Deneen wanted to craft a solution that fit her clinic, her staff, and her patient.

How Family and Friends Reacted

The Hebrew word, "Hineini" means "I am here." It captures the impor-tance of responsiveness, showing up, being personally accountable. "Hineini" describes my family and friends. Days after that awful weekend spent telling everyone about our sad news, my sisters (all out-of-town) sent a beautiful pair of earrings. They almost sent a nightgown, but decided instead on the earrings because they wanted to add cheer to my going "out and about" rather than help me prepare for the occasional idle days in bed. Our son Michael is best friends with Ben Falik. Ben and Ben's father, Aoe Falik, (on behalf of his wife Deborah and family) stopped by that weekend with a beautifully framed photo of Michael and Ben, as well as lots of little goodies from Northern Michigan. Michael was working that summer as a camp counselor in Wisconsin. The camp directors, Roger and Judy Wallenstein, offered to retrieve Michael from a wilderness trip and send him home for a weekend. We didn't take them up on the offer, but the gesture was comforting nonetheless. Instead, Michael learned of the news from Judy, and then he called us to talk some more. Our older son, Brian, and his girlfriend (now wife), Joanna, live in Boston. They were so devastated by our initial conversation that they called Joanna's parents who alerted us to the need to call the kids back to further reassure them. An oncologist I used to work with called to offer his personal support, and then he sent a beautiful plant. Actually, our house had at least one bouquet of fresh flowers or new plant from the first week of my diagnosis to the very last day of my treatment.

My husband and I had been married for almost 29 years when I was diag-nosed, and like most couples had almost unconsciously fallen into a division of labor that suited our temperaments and talents. Now, without any discussion, Hal recognized the need to break out of our traditional habits and take charge of communicating with the outside world. I preferred to retreat periodically, finding that quiet helped calm my anxieties, while conversations tended to stir the emotions. Hal seemed so capable in his new role as "social director" and "personal protector" that I almost forgot how much he was suffering until his secretary, Mary Rutkoske, commented on how shocking it was to see Hal cry at work.

Early on, I tried to spare Hal the need to take off work for my doctor's appointments and chemotherapy treatments by asking some of my friends to accompany me. He quietly but firmly announced that I could make any arrangements I wanted to, but that he was planning to be there for everything. There were times when I overreacted to his lighthearted comments, bursting into tears at his innocent observations about my grocery list or weekend plans. Once Hal thought it would be "good for me" to make a turkey for an injured friend. Since I love to cook and Hal loves to barbeque, he thought this activity would be a great way to keep me involved. I reluctantly agreed, but I found standing on my feet for the time it took to prepare not one, but two (!) turkeys, way too tiring. I remember feeling angry that Hal so underestimated the depth of my fatigue. In reality, I know this lack of energy is almost impossible to convey to others. It's a symptom much written about, difficult to see, and for which there are only partial remedies.

There were other times when we both lay awake all night contemplating worst case scenarios that neither told the other about until the next day. We held onto each other, and were aware of the stream of salt water pouring onto the pillows, but lacked the fortitude to put words into feelings in the dark of night. One such instance was when a CAT scan identified lesions on my liver that could have been benign cysts or evidence of metastasis. I sobbed out loud, "I'd really rather not die young," and then silently spent the night envisioning the outcomes of slow death (chemotherapy working for a time, with multiple relapses) versus quick death (immediate tumor progression despite chemotherapy). Hal's nightmarish thoughts focused on what he might ask me to do (journaling, videos, writing obituaries ahead of time) to help our family prepare for my death. As soon as Dr. B. called us with the good news (benign cysts), we faced each other and confessed almost simultaneously, "I'll tell you what I was thinking if you'll tell me what you were thinking."

As soon as people got the news, they started showing up on our doorstep with the three ingredients for visiting the sick (known in Hebrew as Bikur Cholim): encouragement, practical assistance, and prayer. "Hineini!: I am here, and I'm coming!" At first, we had to keep both our cell phones on in addition to our two home telephone lines to handle all the calls. Upon hearing the news, my friend Naomi Pinchuk hung up the phone mid-sentence and drove over, only to apologize for intruding and offer to go immediately away. Believe me, I was so thankful to sit face-to-face with her that afternoon. At different times each one of my three sisters, two of my college roommates, and another friend flew in to help and to offer encouragement. When I wanted to attend services for my father's yartzheit (anniversary of his death) the day after my first chemotherapy treatment, my friend Roberta insisted that I stop first at her house for a homemade smoothie to ensure that I'd be properly hydrated (and so I could receive a dose of her very good nurse/friendship advice).

My sister Lynn took me out for my first foray into wig shopping. I later learned to laugh at what seemed like a very unfunny situation at the time. Up until that day, I believed I had brown hair, just like I still believe I'm a young woman. Surprise! Every time I selected an acceptable wig and chose the color swatch that most closely matched my hair color, the shop proprietor would painstakingly and somewhat pityingly inform me that the wig wasn't available in that color. "There's really no call for it, dear, so the manufacturing companies don't supply them in that color." What color am I talking about? That mixture of gray/brown that is undyed aging hair. That's right, there are wigs in every color except for those of us who actually wear our own natural color. My college-age friend Judith Horwitz accompanied me for the first wig trimming, and my friend Laurie Pappas (who, in a symbolic gesture, had already delivered three boxes of Life cereal to the house) stayed with me during the 4-hour procedure of getting my head shaved and my wig completely fitted.

Some Russian friends, believing caviar and ginger posses healing powers, delivered these delicacies in surprising abundance. Another friend, Tanya Rubinstein, sent a book of prayers from Germany. My father-in-law in Maryland began calling every Sunday at 12:30 P.M. (after the morning news shows and before the all-important TV sports). My former boss, Richard Preisman, a psychiatrist with a dry wit and a cancer survivor himself, called with advice as well as a knowledgeable listening ear. At times all he uttered were a string of "yeses and mmm-hmms," and at other times he directed, "Don't think of this now. Deal with that later." Our Rabbi called, and called again.

When my counts plummeted 2 weeks after the first chemotherapy, and it looked like I might not be allowed to go to the synagogue for Rosh Hashanah, my friend Debra offered to come to our home with a shofar blower (the ram's horn traditionally sounded at the Jewish New Year). Happily, my counts rose just in time for the arrival of my sisters, brother-in-law, and children, all of whom flew in so we could be together for the start of the Jewish New Year. My sister Joan arrived a few days before Rosh Hashanah to help prepare the big meal, only to find that she had to go shopping alone while I remained housebound, waiting for my counts to improve. Undaunted, she remained after the holiday to accompany Hal and me to the second chemotherapy treatment.

Two days after every chemotherapy treatment my friends Naomi Pinchuk, Debra Darvick, and Sara Zwickl brought lunch. They ate, and I tried to. Following lunch, we usually talked for a bit. Sometimes Debra would read drafts from the book she was writing. After this brief visit, I took a nap, now a daily (sometimes twice daily) necessity.

Many friends sent flowers, books, and poems. They took me for walks in beautiful parks or just little strolls around the neighborhood. From the very beginning we ate our way through the terror by having one picnic after another. It became a running joke with our out-of-town callers. "Whom are you having for dinner tonight?" they'd inquire. Hal called the dinners "little shivas" (traditionally a gathering of friends after a loved one dies), not because we were focused on dying, but because we were being helped, through the presence of others, to mourn our losses and move forward with living.

As the days unfolded into weeks, a rather odd transition occurred. The more help I received, the more I appreciated the soothing effect of being nurtured. Usually known for my independence, I began to revel in the sense of security that came from surrendering my care to others. This transition to "receiver" from "giver" was undoubtedly fostered by a change in the way friends approached me. People, beginning with my younger sisters, started calling me "sweetie," and speaking to me more slowly than before. Maybe they were able to discern something about my mental processes that I hadn't noticed. In any case, who wouldn't regress a little if one's peers suddenly began addressing them as "sweetie"?!

And the cards, oh my, the steady stream of cards—one, from a former Jesuit Priest and current hospice nurse talked about Greek philosophy. Many were hysterically irreverent. Here are just a few examples:

Two e-mails from Ken Grunow, Hospice Nurse

Dear Wendy,
    I was so sorry to hear of your illness . . . When Sondra spoke about it, she mentioned her own take, "Aw, shit!" My "take," not nearly so pithy, was to be reminded of a course I took many years ago (the fall of Troy, as related in the Aeneid). The professor pointed out Virgil's observation that the excellence and achievements of the best citizens of Troy did not save them from the sword. I have been reminded of that many times since, as I have heard of good, good people suffering outrageous misfortunes no one should have to face, let alone those who are trying to bring help to others and good to the world. What inspires, however, is the courage and persistence of so many who, knowing the risks, injustices, and cruelties of life, continue to do good work in the very teeth of adversity.

Dear Wendy,
    So here I am, asking a favorite question. How's life? It is a standard form of greeting in Ghana, where I had the privilege of teaching back in the 70's . . . I like the greeting because it suggests (to my mind, anyway), a hint of the "flavor" of living, how it is currently tasting . . . My hope is that, underneath it all, life still tastes good (but this may be exactly the wrong question at this time. If so, sorry).
    I was also thinking this morning of an idea I heard about while I was doing some adult ed courses . . . My advisor was "big" on the notion of the "wounded healer." He argued that all of us, if we are trying to do any good on this earth, are wounded healers, people coping with our own shortcomings, hurts and injuries, mistakes, disappointments—unhealed wounds even while we are trying to help others.

E-mail from Helen Carvell, friend and retired nurse

Wendy—How could you have an ANC (absolute neutrophil count) of 100? [Counts below 500 place the individual at serious risk of infection.] Call them back; tell them who you are. You have to have 1000 so you can go in and heal the sick. Duh. Of course a Republican wouldn't know that.

From the many greeting cards (*italicized portions are the sender's comments*):

Four greeting cards from Lynn Axelroth, my sister:

Card with a kitten and duck on the cover. Message: *This is too crazy to make any sense of—so we can't and don't. We just know we love you.*
  Card with a dog in a coat, hat, and mittens. Message: What's more important—that you don't catch cold or that people don't laugh at you? . . . *We hope there's no need for a mask, but if there is, we promise not to laugh AT you. But we hope there WILL be a lot of laughing.*
  Card with a CEO-type giving instructions to an attack dog: Message: I want you to go to the Personnel Director and bite him, then to Sales and bite Hempstead and Beasley, then trot on down to the Bookkeeper . . . *Whatever you say, whatever you need.*
  Card with muffin tins on the cover: Message: Does anyone really know the muffin man?

Three notes from Joan Axelroth, my sister:

Card with a woman in leather bindings. Message: Some mornings it just doesn't seem worth it to gnaw through the leather straps . . . *On those mornings, stay in bed.*
  Greeting card with a woman holding her head as if she has a headache. Message: Having a family is like having a bowling alley installed in your brain . . . *Just tell us when you need a break and we'll try to bowl more quietly.*

This message came on pretty stationery:

Dear Wend,
  Thanks for the birthday card with the sweetest of messages.
  Thanks for the birthday card from you and Hal with the funniest of kitties on the cover.
  Thanks for the Chanukah card with thank yous listing every single thing (and then some) anyone has done . . . When did you find the time to make such a list! Very funny . . . even though it was the least we could have done and called for no special mention.
  Thanks for the Edna St. Vincent Millay biography.
  Thanks for you [*sic*] birthday call and conversation.
  Did I miss anything? Oh, yeah—thanks for hanging in there and getting through the year with grace and humor (almost always) so we can all be together to face another.

My cancer treatments ended in the winter. The following summer our good friends Margaret Jordan and Michael Parker planted a beautiful tree of life in our backyard.

THE SURGICAL OPERATION

"Chance favors the prepared mind." Quoting Louis Pasteur, Dr. N. discussed the knowns and unknowns of treating early stage breast cancer. Dr. N. shares Louis Pasteur's attitude toward science even in his everyday surgical work.

Patients think of surgery as totally mystifying, but in reality, there's a bit of the routine in all clinical practice. What is special about Dr. N. and surgeons like him is that they never allow prior mastery to supplant inquisitiveness and critical thought. One may find the expected 100 procedures in a row, and on the 101st need to make an adjustment for the unexpected. This difficult task confronts most of us when driving for extended periods on quiet roads or when performing repetitive tasks. I appreciated having a thinking surgeon, not just "smart enough" but always striving to improve his skills, and always alert for the unexpected. I also appreciated being the patient of someone who respected me, liked me, and seemed to *want* to take care of me. Even though no one should choose "niceness" over surgical skills, rapport does matter not only for its psychological merits, but also because necessary doctor/patient communication is impeded when rapport is lacking.

When Dr. N. asked me to participate in a clinical study that required bilateral bone marrow biopsies during surgery, I didn't hesitate because I believed he wouldn't ask me to do something unreasonable or overly burdensome. When he insisted on calling the procedure a partial mastectomy instead of a lumpectomy, I actually felt that he respected the kind of visual defect and long-term sequelae such an operation creates for the patient. I can tell you now (but did not realize then) that a lumpectomy is far, far different from an excisional biopsy. When my first surgery didn't produce so-called "clean" (tumor free) margins, I trusted that Dr. N. made the best surgical decisions he could have in the OR, and that my second surgery was necessary because of the limits of science, not because he "missed something" that others could have found. To demonstrate just how "dense" my tissue actually is, Dr. N. said that even a flat plate x-ray of the excised tumor couldn't identify where the tumor ended and normal tissue began. My "denseness" has become a family joke, and is a term sometimes used to refer to my cognitive processes rather than my cellular tissue whenever I do something a bit goofy (as I have been known to do from time to time).

One bit of advice for OR staff: let the patient's family remain with her during the entire pre-op experience *if* the patient wishes. What's the point of sending the spouse to the waiting room during the first few minutes of the patient's surrendering street clothes for a hospital gown and answering the nurse's assessment questions? The beginning of any experience is when the patient is most anxious, and would benefit the most from the presence of a loved one. That I *can* do without my husband doesn't mean I should *have* to. That the nurses are as kind as can be doesn't mean they can replace the beneficial support of a relative or friend. This is a pet peeve of mine that I will refer to again in this chapter. I much prefer the salve of human presence (sometimes denied) to the effect of sedating drugs (always freely offered). Besides, a relative's presence is not solely for the benefit of the patient. My husband is consoled by seeing in real time what is actually happening. He wants to "be there," not just hear about it. Remember, what is totally routine and unremarkable for staff is poignantly meaningful to patients and families.

One of many "thank-yous" due to the OR staff: Thanks for aggressively treating my post-op pain. I awoke whispering, "It hurts, it hurts, it hurts," as I experienced a very localized, intense, burning sensation. A bit of IV morphine was followed soon with the question, "How are you doing now?" Ah, assessment and timely reassessment, something I emphasize when teaching clinicians how to manage pain. Another little dose of morphine and I was alert and totally comfortable. I didn't think anyone knew I was a pain management expert, but I remember feeling relieved that I didn't have to battle my way to good pain relief. Then came the funny part—the house officer elicited my advice about discharge analgesics, which I gladly volunteered as I apologized for being too groggy to explain the principles behind my recommendations. Someone must have "squealed." He obviously knew I was "in the business," and I really appreciated his attempt to include my input in the treatment plan.

One amusing thing about Dr. N.'s genuine concern for me: No matter how many times he read the pathology report, or was reminded of the results by me, he could not accept that my tumor was ER (−). He so did not want me to have to endure a course of chemotherapy, that he kept discussing, and later handing me articles about chemotherapy's lack of benefit for small ER (+) tumors. His personal anguish was so endearing, even though I realized all along that chemotherapy was the appropriate course of action. I knew Dr. N. wasn't trying to preempt my oncologist's advice. He just wanted my life to be less burdensome, and he feared for the effects of chemotherapy on intellect, a capacity both of us highly value.

I noticed another peculiar little tension that occurred during pre- and post-op office visits. I was *so* satisfied with the outcome of the surgery and with the personal care I received from Dr. N. and nurses Milica Kay, R.N., and Paula Robinson, R.N., Yet, I felt it was my duty to report all symptoms so that the experts could triage the relevant from the irrelevant. However, there were times when I felt (not because of anything the staff communicated, but only because of my own insecurities) that reporting symptoms was tantamount to complaining. How could a person whose care had been so elegant, whose symptoms were so minimal, and whose prognosis was so good, how could such a person complain? I feared that reporting symptoms might demonstrate lack of gratitude, but I was too afraid not to report. This inner tension is the stuff for a psychiatrist's couch, or at least a heart-to-heart talk with a friend over lunch. I expect that most patients experience this conflict at one time or another. Certainly, many of my patients have spoken of it in their own way.

Another little ongoing tension might be peculiar to Dr. N.'s style of interaction and my style of patient behavior, although I suspect we both have some brethren out there who react similarly. Dr. N. and I have much in common and know each other's children, so we spend the first few minutes of each examination in social conversation. I've had so many examinations over the years that my mind usually floats off to some distant place, like a participant-observer, decreasing embarrassment and any of the unpleasant aspects of medical treatment. This works fine when all I have to do is passively follow commands like

"Lift your arm," or "Take a deep breath." Daydreaming doesn't work so well for responding to nuanced questions like, "Is there any difference in sensation in this spot versus that spot?" For that you have to concentrate. There's no reason that Dr. N. or any of my physicians should have known that I'm not really paying attention when they examine me, but I can tell you that it's very jarring trying to respond to questions when one is temporarily very distant from one's body. I don't want this to sound freakish. It's a subtle, and rather brief state of being. Nonetheless, I have found myself occasionally tongue-tied trying to bring my focus back fast enough to answer questions in real time. Once I stalled by saying, "Would you like me to concentrate?" hoping I could bring myself to full alertness in time for the next probing question. "Please," he said politely.

Little bits of advice: So glad I bought two sports bras before surgery. They helped immediately post-op and all the way through radiation therapy. Blue dye (used to identify the sentinel node) creates a weird and almost humorous change in the appearance of the affected breast. Laughing is better than crying. No matter how many health care degrees one has, there is no substitute for expert guidance when dealing with bandages and wounds. The physical sensations of healing can add to the fears of missed disease even when one knows intellectually that this is a highly unlikely prospect. These sensations are distracting because of their novelty, sudden onset, negative effect on sleep, painfulness or any combination of the above. All of the sensations were manageable, but it did help to have medical assurance as to their etiology and nonserious significance. Paraphrasing Victor Frankl, one who knows the "why" can bear almost any "how." It was a little disconcerting to hear, "I don't know why you're experiencing this," and more rarely, "You shouldn't be having this problem."

After the surgery and radiation treatments, for example, my arm on the surgical side kept going numb, or at best, felt like it was heavy and bruised even though it didn't appear to be swollen. This occurred day and night, but was especially disruptive during the night because it interrupted my sleep about every hour. No one knew why I experienced these symptoms with just two limited surgeries, a sentinel lymph node biopsy and radiation. The lack of an etiology frightened me. Had I suddenly become psychosomatic (experiencing physical symptoms as a substitute for emotions)? Could an undiagnosed injury or worse, an undetected cancer, explain my plight? Even though I "shouldn't" have had this problem, Dr. B. took a chance and referred me to the lymphedema clinic where I learned to massage and bandage my arm. Several days after applying the bandages, I got a good night's sleep. I still don't know what the explanation is for this problem, but when it occurs, now I know what to do. I've since had a patient report the same constellation of symptoms, and I've heard a lecture about this underdiagnosed syndrome at an Oncology Nursing Society meeting. That's some comfort that I haven't lost my senses. I'm curious about the etiology, but pleased to have a workable remedy. I never use the bandages in public now. The symptoms still interrupt my sleep every night, but as I said to a friend recently, my "bristle response" has decreased, so the symptoms are no longer as upsetting as they once were.

CHEMOTHERAPY

It's so doable, but so unfun. That about sums up chemotherapy. Here are some of the things that helped make the treatments bearable: going to each session with my husband and a friend or family member; being warmly welcomed by the staff who treat everyone like a temporary member of the family; having options for treating nausea so that when one medication failed to control those iggy feelings, another could be tried; frequent naps; journaling; simple activities that didn't tax the brain.

Here's something that didn't help: scheduling my port placement for the same day as my first chemotherapy treatment. Cognizant of the wear and tear of numerous medical appointments on newly diagnosed patients, the clinic staff encouraged me to arrange for placement of a central venous access device (port) the morning of my first chemotherapy treatment. Most people do it this way, but I think we should reconsider the practice. The medication used to achieve what's known as "conscious sedation," for the port placement caused extreme nausea, and then rendered me unarousable for several hours. I do not remember arriving in the chemotherapy room, nor do I recall the educational video that the nurse says she showed me. Later, people joked about how neat it was that I got to sleep through my entire first treatment. Sounds good on paper, but this is actually counterproductive for the patient. I needed to get oriented to this whole new routine, but couldn't because I was unconscious. Indeed, there is a state of semiarousal that is often mistaken for wakefulness when the individual, with eyes completely open, can respond to simple commands, but is unable to think clearly or remember what is being said. I teach this concept to trainees all the time, but wasn't coherent enough to communicate the relevant points to the health care team that afternoon. I remember my Nurse Practitioner friend, Cathy Baldy, helping me onto the bedside commode, and my saying to her, "I never thought I'd be doing this with you, Cathy." I remember the nurse (an excellent and kind oncology nurse) telling me several times, "but I told you that already," or "that was covered in the video," and thinking to myself in a fog, "What is she talking about?" Being oversedated is different from being calm. Being sedated is disorienting, perplexing, and is actually anxiety provoking. Of course, individuals vary in their sensitivity to sedatives, but many of my patients have reported similar reactions to this scenario. I wonder if it might not be better to offer patients a choice about the timing of their port placement, describing the range of responses to the procedure and their potential effects on the first chemotherapy experience.

I developed a little pattern for managing both chemotherapy treatment days and the weeks between treatments. For the uninitiated, patients usually feel their best the day of treatment because their blood counts have recovered from the previous chemotherapy, and they're reasonably well rested. Chemotherapy changes all that, cycling the patient through a pattern of increasing and then subsiding symptoms until the next chemotherapy comes due. Happily, each treatment day turned into a big social event for us because different colleagues stopped in to say hello and chat while the IV chemotherapy did its little job. Once, Dr. L., one of the newer oncologists I had never met, asked if she could introduce herself to me because she wanted to thank me for all that I had done for her patients. What a touching and affirming gesture! Hal and I told ourselves that taking pictures of the staff and "the scene" would help our sons grasp the goings on. In truth, I think the act of picture taking (pictures we've rarely looked at since) helped my husband and me come to terms with our present reality.

On the drive home from chemotherapy we'd pick up a movie and spend the evening stretched out on the couch usually with the friend or family member who accompanied us to chemo that day. I didn't always remain awake until the end of the movie, but watching helped us maintain a relaxed atmosphere. I learned not to try to eat that first night, but did take in enough fluids to keep the plumbing working. We always called our sons, my sisters, and Hal's father to assure our support team that once again, everything was OK.

The day after chemo was a totally down day consisting of awakening from bed only in order to nap on the couch on and off most of the day, in order to go upstairs again and go to bed. It was on those days that I wrote in my journal, relished opening greeting cards, read (but not always answered) emails, and listened to (but not always returned) phone calls. The "Bikur Cholim" Wednesday lunch bunch previously described filled day 2 with a little variety that included both lighthearted banter and serious "women talk." All three of the women took time out from their jobs and family obligations to make the afternoon an incredibly pleasant one. On Thursday (day 3 after chemo) I returned to work, seasick and fatigued. My colleagues and my family helped me meet this challenge and truly made it possible for me to continue working.

We didn't do much the first two weekends after treatment. However, Hal always planned a fun activity for the third weekend when I was in a better position to be sociable and enjoy the food that inevitably accompanies our activities. Bless our friends for tolerating these abbreviated outings as well as my occasionally odd behavior. Already perimenopausal at the time of my diagnosis, I constantly struggled with a kind of temperature dysregulation that one could not solve entirely by dressing in layers. When faced with the prospect of cooling down or passing out, it's amazing how shameless one can become. Jackets were tossed off revealing sleeveless camisoles and "old lady arms" never meant for public view. There were times when I excused myself from the dining table of fancy restaurants to slip off my pantyhose in the ladies room, and return to the table with my bare feet in good heels. At other times, I cooled down by removing the hat from my bald, bald head. I usually asked the indulgence of our dinner companions, and not a one ever flinched. It was comforting to know that Hal really liked my bald look, and in a strange kind of way, I also enjoyed this throwback to our hippy days—thin face, cool earrings, edgy appearance. Cancer entitles one to a small range of behaviors that are normally taboo. I tried not to take advantage of this weird "perk," although giving in once in a while helped me function. I knew then, and believe now, however, that I'd trade all the perks that come with being ill for never having been sick at all.

My dentist, Dr. F., provided me with a list of oral hygiene supplies to help prevent and/or treat the mouth sores and dental problems that sometimes occur when a person's immune system is suppressed. I grumbled about spending yet more money on cancer, but found his recommendations for electric toothbrush, toothpaste, fluoride rinse, gum balm, and mouthwash products all quite useful, and have since passed this list along to others. My oncologist and the chemo nurses really seemed to want to know what was working and what wasn't, and always had suggestions for new things to try to deal with any annoying symptoms.

The chemo nurses and my social worker friends knew about the importance of mirth during these weeks of perpetual sickness and drudgery. With Sherry Perry, R.N., as instigator and party planner, they surprised me on the last day of chemotherapy with a graduation certificate, nonalcoholic champagne (red and white), a king-size comb for my bald head, goofy glasses, and a giant cake. I have always believed that part of my job is to make *all* of my patients VIPs no matter their background. Now my friends made me the VIP.

RADIATION THERAPY

For those of us who completed surgery and chemotherapy prior to radiation treatment, radiation therapy represents quite an important milestone. There is the elation of being almost finished with cancer treatment, and the despair of having to face another 6 or 7 weeks of medical treatments. The good news is that the fatigue that results from radiation therapy is not as all consuming as the symptoms that often accompany chemotherapy. It's true that it takes much longer to drive to, undress for, and then dress again after treatment than it does to receive the actual radiation therapy. But there's so much more to treatment than the actual minutes spent receiving one or another form of radiation beam.

In order to receive external beam radiation (the most common form of radiation treatment for breast cancer patients), a simulation must be performed to help the radiation oncologist and dosimetrist plan the exact locations and amounts of treatment that would give the patient the greatest benefit and the least side effects—another example of the art and science of medicine. The simulation room looks exactly like the treatment room. However, during simulation, x-rays are taken, some discussion occurs among physician, dosimetrist and techs, and body tattoos are injected—all in preparation for the series of radiation treatments that follow. My husband wanted to be present for the

simulation, but was told this was impossible. The reasons given weren't logical, so just as in the discourse on whole breast ultrasound or the operating
room edicts on patient's visitors, I persisted in challenging the rationale. We
always tell patients to voice their concerns and advocate for change, but as
an employee *and* a patient, I was wary of causing a stir. My professional role
includes supporting colleagues, not just patients. Strong-willed by nature, I'm
also known for my kindness and ability to easily establish rapport. I wanted
to earn the prize for being the easiest patient to care for, not the most difficult. There was a moment in the simulation room that challenged my ability
to find common ground, maintain my equanimity, and continue in the "good
patient" role. While I was prone on the simulation table, an extremely efficient and bright staff member standing at the foot of the table grabbed my
ankles, leaned over me, and appealed to my position as colleague and hospital
representative.

"Look, she said sternly, "I'm sure in *your* territory, it's *your* job to enforce
the rules."

I retorted, "In *my* territory, it's *my* job to ensure that the needs of the patients,
families, and staff are all met."

"Let him stay," uttered the exasperated doctor.

Hal remained quietly tucked into an out-of-the way corner of the room. We
both appreciated his presence, and I have since tried to explain how important a
first experience is to a patient and spouse. Offering family members permission
to witness the second episode in the treatment room (technically the first actual
treatment), is no substitute for being there at the beginning when the whole
experience is unfamiliar. I still regret this unpleasant entree to my relationship
with the radiation oncology staff, but I am impressed with everyone's ability to
move beyond that moment to achieve the excellent care that was everyone's
goal from the start. I tell this story, not because I relish exposing my weaknesses
or the rare moments in our health care system when care is more rote than
customer service driven. I tell this story to emphasize that we can live in an
imperfect world, and still do very, very well. We live with imperfection, but it
takes all of us—patients, families, and health care professionals alike—to help
make things better. Conflict may not be pleasant, but it's probably unavoidable.
Long established routines deserve to be questioned. Through carefully handled
dissent we can learn things—about ourselves, each other, and the whole health
care delivery system.

Here's something else I learned that I might not have realized had I only
been on the health care side of things: Once in place on the treatment table,
the gigantic room felt just like "my" room for the few minutes I was assigned
to it every day. If you've ever been hospitalized, you know how it feels when
staff or visitors enter your patient room without knocking, even though they
have legitimate business there. Well, patients on a radiation treatment table
are cautioned to remain motionless once in position on the treatment table to
preserve the integrity of the treatment plan and avoid injury to themselves. The
radiation oncology techs' highly skilled and clear instructions communicated

both a sense of security and the importance of following these very sensible rules. The techs always announced their intentions to enter the room through an intercom or by calling into the room from the doorway. In contrast, other staff members thought it was acceptable to enter the room while treatment was in progress without alerting me first. Remember, the patient can hear but cannot see much besides the radiation equipment while wedged into position. One lies on the table exposed from the waist up. The staff's explanations for not announcing themselves were that they didn't want me to move in response to their vocal pronouncements. In truth, I almost bolted upright the first time I heard footsteps in the room and didn't know who was there. Unexpected entrances feel like disrespectful, disturbing intrusions, while preannounced visits add to one's sense of comfort and security.

Toward the end of radiation therapy it's not unusual to experience a little skin breakdown—something like a bad sunburn. Kudos to Karen Kloustin, R.N., Radiation Oncology Nurse, who suggested balms and protective padding to ease the pain, decrease irritation, and promote healing. Dr. B. volunteered another helpful remedy in the form of a topical medication. I appreciated not only the remedies, but also the interest both individuals demonstrated in easing what was certainly a low-level and temporary problem. Both Ms. Kloustin and Dr. B. indicated that no one should have to endure unnecessary discomfort, and seemed to take pride in solving whatever problems they could.

My radiation treatments ended just before the New Year. My husband, Hal, son Brian and his girlfriend Joanna, son Michael and his best friend Ben, and I took off for Toronto. Nothing like enjoying the *Lion King*, China Town, and museums with those nearest and dearest to help make one feel whole again.

How I Was Able to Work during My Treatments

Like most things in life, "ability to work" has inextricably intertwined psychological, physical, and environmental components. I did work during treatment, but in a modified way.

Within 2 days of my diagnosis, Dr. E., a psychologist on our Consultation-Liaison Psychiatry service, called me to express her concern, and to offer a plan she devised for covering my patients and keeping me in touch with work. Her concern for the service, for patients, and for me personally, as well as Anne's characteristic attention to detail, eased the transition from workaholic to my new status as partly functioning colleague.

Anne and the secretaries rearranged patient schedules. Anne saw some individuals who required immediate attention, and Dr. K., another C-L psychologist, took over the care of most new inpatient consults. Anne brought mail home, drove me to work during short periods when I wasn't permitted to drive, and generally kept me informed. My secretaries, Mary Cantu and Cynthia Maxie, always protective and loyal, took on an even more active triage role, delivering essential messages, and handing off what they could to other staff. I decided to continue seeing all my current outpatients, but for 5 months accepted no new patients, and saw only a few inpatients. I also used vacation time to give me an extra day off per week, which meant that my part-time position fell from three 12-hour days to two 8-hour days.

What made work challenging was the show-stopping fatigue and intermittent periods of nausea that permeated my life throughout treatment. I truly wanted to pull my weight as a colleague, and was (still am) conscious of appearing as "damaged goods." It's possible to hide most of what one is experiencing, but that seemed almost disrespectful to the plight of cancer patients in general, a population for whom I consider myself an advocate. Maintaining the façade of a "happy, well-adjusted cancer patient" is not only disingenuous, but also adds to one's exhaustion. Realistically, my troubles paled in comparison to many others'. This perspective made it possible to confine my complaints to a few "inner circle" family and friends. A psychiatrist I knew asked me how I was faring. I mused, "if only I could refer myself to myself, I think I'd be in much better shape." That understated way of acknowledging the down times helped me cope, even though I never did seek formal outside professional assistance. It's hard to appear upbeat when one can't remember what it feels like to feel well. It's hard to know how long to maintain the protective cocoon of modified work expectations—fearing both the inability to meet the challenges of a full load and the dangers that come with losing one's "relevance" in a competitive workforce.

As for the ever-present fatigue . . . I usually took a short nap on my itty-bitty office couch at the end of the day just so I could garner the strength to walk to the parking lot and drive home. Honestly, some days I just looked at my legs and out loud commanded them to move. Once home, my husband always greeted me at the door to carry in my brief case and whatever other paraphernalia I needed to bring in from the car. Some days he even treated me by driving me to and from work, offering his good company, and helping me to preserve my diminished energy reserve. The wheels of my mind ground slowly round while the muscles of my limbs resisted activity, but with limited expectations, both functioned. Believe me, I checked and double-checked my work to make sure I was delivering the same safe, high-quality care I gave my patients prior to my diagnosis. To work, I had to forgo all other activities. Work days consisted solely of work and sleep.

All of my patients deserve credit, too. Though they must remain anonymous to you, the reader, I hope I have managed to personally thank everyone who put up with not only rescheduled appointments, but also the anxiety that comes from working with a physically ill therapist. As my colleagues predicted, most patients responded well to this new, but unfortunate bond—a shared cancer diagnosis and many shared symptoms. Some of my long-term patients seemed to relish the opportunity to nurture me as I had nurtured them. "Nothing wrong with equalizing reciprocity in mature relationships," I told myself. However, for therapy to be beneficial, it's critical that the focus remain on the patient—their concerns, their struggles, their experiences. I consciously avoided gratuitous comparisons between patients' stories and my own, never wanting to present myself as "the standard," and always wary of hampering patients' expressions whose private worries might be totally different from my own.

I informed all of the patients I saw during my treatment of my diagnosis, though I provided few details unless specifically asked. As the distance from treatment increased, and my appearance returned to my "normal" just-shy-of-frumpy, middle-aged (gasp!), short woman, I stopped disclosing my diagnosis unless it was clearly part of a therapeutic intervention. Even then, I tended to wait until after several therapy sessions to reveal any personal information so that patients could first establish their counseling priorities, their perspectives, and their style of interacting. I had no idea that a few well-intentioned staff members were divulging my health history until some new patients posed questions at the end of their first session that went something like this:

Patient: "How do you do it?"

Wendy: "Do what?" (Expecting to hear, "take care of so many ill people . . . see so many cancer patients," or something similar.)

Patient: "You know."

Wendy: "Please tell me."

Patient: "You're a cancer patient, aren't you? They (nurse, doctor, etc.) told me you had cancer too."

The first time I heard this, I couldn't believe my ears. By the third time, I knew I had to do something. My dear, sweet colleagues feel so at ease with me, that they thought it would be "OK" and even a good idea to include my health history as an added endorsement during the referral process. Apparently, these few individuals were telling patients something like, "You'll really like her. She's a cancer patient too." It's true that disclosing another's health data constitutes a legal breech, but honestly, I can understand how even thinking health care professionals might have (incorrectly) given this situation exempt status. They know me as an open person, they feel comfortable with me, and most importantly, these individuals would do *anything*, absolutely anything to help their patients. So, after recovering from the shock of these revelations, I tried to devise a way of fixing the leaks in an educational, rather than a punitive manner. Through a group meeting with staff, conversations with mid-level administrators, and a few face-to-face conversations with colleagues I tried to explain the key reasons for maintaining my privacy:

1. Referrals were being made to me on the basis of my credentials and skills as a therapist, and not because of my cancer diagnosis. In fact, I'd worked successfully in this field for 20 years before having cancer. There didn't seem to be any barrier to care that these revelations would overcome.

2. Self-disclosure is a therapeutic intervention that must serve the patient, making it important for *me*, not the staff, to determine what personal information to reveal and when to reveal it. I was glad to talk about my illness when this conversation could truly benefit the patient.

3. I greatly valued my therapeutic relationship with all the staff caring for me, and wanted to feel comfortable continuing our open interactions, trusting that

the staff would treat the information they had as a sacred trust. Operating from this assumption, I could then invite all staff members to privately pose any question they wished, at any time now or in the future. I would do the best I could to answer as long as I knew they would hold the information in confidence.
4. Finally, I had to do some mental maneuvering to succeed as a therapist with "cancer patient" being now a permanent aspect of my identity. Like many of my colleagues, I repeatedly receive the "great grief cry" that Rainer Maria Rilke so aptly describes. I can use my own physical symptoms and psychological anxieties to better inform my work as a therapist, but I cannot indulge these feelings in a way that could diminish my strength as a caregiver. I have to remain focused and robust at work, and that means containing some of my personal insecurities while ministering to patients and colleagues.

As it turns out, this "meeting of the minds" served to strengthen collegial relationships, and helped me clarify for myself the balancing act required in this now permanent dual role. I'm indebted to Deneen Ihlenfeldt, R.N., for inviting me to speak with her staff, and to the other administrators and clinicians who willingly, openly and nondefensively discussed these issues with me.

My Spiritual Connection

The year after completing treatment, our Rabbi asked me to give a Yom Kippur address on the meaning that Judaism had during my illness. The honor of addressing our congregation on the most solemn afternoon of the Hebrew calendar, our Day of Atonement, moved me to engage in some soul-searching reflection that contributed mightily to my healing journey. Rabbi Roman knows that I'm somewhat nontraditional even for a Reform Jew. He knows that my strong connection to Judaism is primarily to its history, its people, its magnificent cultural attributes and beautiful rituals, and its tremendous relevance for daily living, rather than to a focus on a supreme being. He knows this, but invited me to speak anyway. As a result of preparing for the talk, I came away with an even deeper appreciation for Judaism's contribution to building a caring community.

I believe that illness isn't fair or earned or deserved. It isn't punishment. God doesn't make us sick. The Talmud (an authoritative interpretation of ancient oral law) teaches that when the famous Rabbi Yochanan became ill, another Rabbi asked him if man's sufferings are welcome. Rabbi Yochanan replied, "Neither they nor their reward." To put it bluntly, illness isn't a good thing, even when some good comes from the experience.

Of the 613 biblical commandments, 213 are concerned with medical issues. Is healing science or art? Should it be based on concrete knowledge or spiritual remedies? Judaism, with its strong traditions of scientific inquiry (the first clinical trial is described in the book of Daniel) affirms that healing must address both the needs of the body and of the spirit. My health care team, family, and friends truly understood these principles.

Judaism also teaches that patients have a responsibility to seek medical care, to communicate with their caregivers, and to follow through with recommended treatments. I didn't want the "patient role" to consume every aspect of my personhood, but I did (and do) feel some responsibility to approach my patient status as a job. I have to show up on time, prepare, demonstrate tenacity, be flexible, and solve problems—in short, be an active participant in my own care.

Judaism teaches that the preservation of human life takes precedence over all Jewish laws except commandments against adultery, murder, and incest. The Talmud teaches that fear accelerates the pulse and causes abnormal heartbeats. It recognizes the power of human presence to assuage this kind of fear. The Sabbath, for example, is supposed to be a happy time, but it is still acceptable to visit the sick on the Sabbath even if it means experiencing the sadness that naturally accompanies visits with the ill. It's remarkable that most Talmudic guidelines governing visits to the sick focus on meeting the interpersonal and psychological needs of the ill. Authoritative Rabbis were not as concerned with ritual rules in these circumstances as they were with sensitivity to the needs of the suffering. "Enter the room cheerfully," was one such command. "He who visits a sick person removes 1/60th of his illness," states another sage, emphasizing the importance of presence and the dangers of isolation. Visitors to the sick should elicit the patient's preferences for the timing and nature of the sick call thus preserving the patient's sense of autonomy.

Ancient sages even recognized that some well-wishers have more limitations than others. "May I be spared visits from stupid people," is the loose translation of one Rabbi's lament. Some of my friends got a kick out of hearing about the "stupid remark of the week" from people who meant well but mistakenly thought I'd find solace in hearing about how much I'd learn from having a life-threatening illness (true, but not worth the risk), or how this was a wake-up call (as if I had brought the illness upon myself), how my family would benefit from taking care of me (true, but not worth the burden and anxiety), how my knowledge would spare me the anguish of lay persons (psychotherapists have feelings too), or what a relief it was that the tumor was small, because the surgeon must have "gotten it all" (a macroscopic surgical truth, but no guarantee against a fatal recurrence). My guess is that we've all uttered regrettable remarks from time to time. Stupid remarks will occur, but with the right attitude, such remarks can become a source of humor.

Talmudic guidelines instruct that visitors to the sick should help with chores, with meals, and with emotional restoration. Visitors to the sick should pray for the patient's recovery (in the presence of the patient or at another time). These three acts, encouragement, practical assistance, and prayer represent the core requirements of Bikur Cholim, the sick call. "Hineni. I am here." Wonderfully supportive people, each with unique talents, Jew and non-Jew alike, surrounded me during the entire course of my illness. I am forever in their debt, although I know they gave of themselves freely without any expectation other than the personal satisfaction that comes from caring about another.

I definitely favor the steadying force of human presence over stoically endured, but unnecessary bravery or mind-numbing chemical tranquilization. However, there are times when medication, judiciously prescribed, can prevent or treat symptoms that interfere with resilience. Judaism supports the medical relief of symptoms through both human presence and pharmacologic assistance. I've found that combining these approaches can contribute greatly to emotional stability.

One of my favorite Hebrew prayers is the Mi Shebeirach, a prayer both for the ill and for their caregivers. I have always found special meaning in singing the Mi Shebeirach aloud during Sabbath services as I silently pondered my patients and my efforts to ease their distress. Now, as a patient myself, the prayer took on even deeper meaning. Often Hal and I would hold hands as we sang the words. Sometimes, a few tears would drip onto our palms. The English translation is as follows:

> May the Source of strength Who blessed the ones before us
> Help us find the courage to make our lives a blessing, And let us say: Amen.
>
> Bless those in need of healing with r'-fu-a she'-lei-ma
> The renewal of body, the renewal of spirit,
> And let us say: Amen.

Interestingly, there is another traditional prayer for the sick spoken during the Jewish High Holidays, which used to disturb me, but which I (shamefully) did nothing about until I, too, became ill. The prayer, uttered out loud, often standing in front of the congregation, beseeches God to grant healing to the afflicted. One line of the prayer requires the sick person to refer to him/herself as "unworthy." The person who wrote the prayer probably thought of the line as reflecting humility in the presence of an almighty figure. I, on the other hand, always believed that all sufferers deserve to have their burdens lifted. One person is not more deserving than another, nor should there be such a category as "unworthy." That we can't all be healed in the preferred way (totally cured, for example) comes from the limitations of science, not some metaphysical edict. After my diagnosis, I discussed with our Rabbi my concerns that the verbiage of the prayer might cause suffering even as it is meant to relieve a sick person's burdens. He, too, admitted some dissatisfaction with the way the liturgy addressed the concerns of the sick, and has in recent years modified or replaced these types of prayers with much more supportive and affirming messages. Even though I've never believed a supreme being actually decided whether I would live or die, I wanted to be able to express my prayerful desire for healing without making derogatory remarks about myself or the sick. Thank you, Rabbi Roman, for addressing these concerns in a way that reflects ancient Jewish teachings and modern wisdom about sickness and health.

MY BIGGEST FEAR

Absolutely, my biggest fear is "living badly." By this I mean, living with such extreme illness that one's life is reduced to joyless burden for the self and for others. Biology without biography is certainly my greatest fear. Having read about, thought about, and witnessed these issues play out for countless patients (and some relatives), I believe I "know" certain things:

1. One's sense of what's tolerable may change as one's circumstances and expectations change.
2. Despite common themes, each person's viewpoint is unique, and can only be defined by that person.
3. Families can handle more than they think, but that willingness only buffers, but does not relieve families from the anguish of caring for a seriously ill relative.

One of my fears was that well-meaning relatives (especially my sisters) might ask me to carry on longer than I wanted to if things started to go badly. I worried that there might be conflict among very close family members, all trying to help, but each guided by their own strong views of health and illness. I worried about assembling one medical team that could fight like hell to keep me well (being vigilant about prevention and treatment) and still be the same team to accept a palliative approach if that ever became necessary. I wanted one team of individuals who could "do it all," but I know this is asking a lot.

I never worried that my friends or family wouldn't talk with me about serious issues even though the possibility of facing any of them is, thankfully, quite remote. Those close to me are open people. They accept my need for directness, and seem to understand that considering "worst case scenarios" from time-to-time is not inconsistent with remaining hopeful and trying to live a full life.

When the radiologist "saw something" on an early CAT scan, and I faced the possibility of having metastatic (and thus fatal) disease at diagnosis, I cried aloud to my husband, "I'd really rather not die young." It's true. I really do not want to die. I think I have much to offer others, and I just relish life. My children, their loved ones, the unborn grandchildren, travels, study, it's all too grand to consider giving up. I want to be here to enjoy and to help my loved ones for a long, long time. I don't want to die, but most of all, I don't want to live badly. I'm willing to make many compromises, but hope I don't have to. I don't want to promise in advance what I'll find acceptable, and what is too much. When I tell you it's too much, you, whoever you are, should believe me.

MY MOST MEMORABLE EXPERIENCE

We turn to our loved ones for sustenance and rejuvenation as it says in Numbers 11(17),

"And I will take of the spirit which is upon thee, and will put it upon them; and
they shall bear the burden of the people with thee, that thou bear it not thyself alone."

After all the treatments were completed, we had a luncheon for our friends on a Sunday in January. The invitation read: "To Celebrate Friendship and the New Year." We wanted to thank everyone who helped throughout my illness, but there was no hiding the fact that this was a sort of "coming out" or "coming back" party. Our children and their respective girlfriends attended colleges out-of-state and were all back in school at this point. Save for missing them and some other close relatives and friends, the party was the perfect ending to 6 months of fear and drudgery. Our house was filled to overfloating with ebullient friends and an abundance of gourmet food (if I do say so myself). We didn't want this to be just "any" party. Hal and I like to cook (and to eat), so we decided to tackle some new recipes to help communicate, through gastronomic delicacies, just how special our friends are to us. Humorous in retrospect only, the menu overreached our physical and time constraints (especially the 47-step Mexican Lasagna which was a big hit, but has never been tackled since). If it weren't for our friends, Ari and Galina Buman, who came over the day before to help with the kitchen prep, I think we would have been cooking still. I don't know how Ari and Galina figured out that we were drowning in preparations on Saturday, but somehow friends just know.

In some ways, nothing can top the sight of a "force of good"—all those friends—gathered in one spot, all celebrating together. That memory makes me smile whenever I reflect on it, which is often. But, the most memorable experience of all was the surprise letter from our sons. Brian and his now-wife Joanna and Michael and his girlfriend Laurie sent roses and a little note the day before the party. This was a total surprise, and certainly communicated how much they felt a part of things despite their distance. The roses took a place of honor in two vases on the serving table. Unbeknownst to us, there was more to come. Just before dessert we gathered everyone in the living room so Hal and I could offer thanks to the assembled friends. It was then that our friend Naomi Pinchuk asked if she could speak. This is what she said (or, more accurately, read):

Hello everybody. For the next few minutes you will have to pretend that I am either Brian or Michael. I know I can't grow a beard like Michael, nor can I properly explain the principles of quantum dots like Brian, but you will just have to accept that this message is from them.

Unfortunately, neither of us could be here today for this gathering and celebration of health and happiness. First off we would like to extend our deepest gratitude to all of you who went above and beyond to help our Mom and our family through this period in our lives. It was difficult for us to be away at school during most of our Mom's treatments. However, we would always hear about the numerous phone calls checking up on her, or friends reading a book to help pass those difficult times, or offering to be there for the momentous hair shaving day, or even just stopping by to say hello and remind her how much she is loved by all of you. Whatever your involvement, it was not only a tremendous help to our Mom, but it was also a great help to my brother and me knowing that our Mom was in such great hands.

"Of all the things which wisdom provides to make life entirely happy, much the greatest is the possession of friendship." – Epicurus

You have all shown yourselves to be the greatest of friends, and we thank you from the bottom of our hearts.

It would of course be wrong of us to leave out the impact of our Dad over this time. Mom, as the nurse in the family, always knew how to make us feel better when we were sick or uncomfortable. Well, I think Mom can vouch for this: Nobody worked harder to help make each day a little easier than our Dad. He has always been a loving husband and a great father to us.

One of the running jokes throughout these past few months was that Mom "wrote the book on breast cancer." Doctors started giving her pamphlets which she helped to create, and found that "Wendy Goldberg" was the person to go to for cancer patients and their families. Well, we used that source and always found that our Mom was there to answer any questions we had or to reassure us that as a family we would get through everything. She has always been the force that binds our family together. Even during her treatment, Mom came down to Indiana University for a weekend, and just after her final treatment she joined us all for a great weekend in Toronto. She would not allow some silly limitations from the treatment to stop her from joining in on all the family fun. So we want to say thank you, Mom, for helping guide us through these last six months. We love you always and forever. —Brian and Michael

And, I love you. That's you: the family, the friends, the health care professionals, the patients—all of you—for making it possible to thrive during the most challenging and also during the happiest of times.

11

AFTERWARD: "AN ABUNDANCE OF RESILIENCE"

Most breast cancer survivors do not simply return to their previous lives, even after the successful course of treatment. They are changed by what happened to them. While the change may include ongoing anxiety about whether the cancer will return, there is also a more surprising consequence of the disease. Some feel, echoing what Lance Armstrong said about his experience with his cancers that cancer was a difficult experience and acted as a "wake up call," they felt a greater sense of awareness, and some achieved a tranquility they had not previously had.

First, let's listen to what some have to say about the ongoing worries. Hardeep said bluntly, "Even today, mammograms/checkups are very anxiety provoking, causing fear, depression." And even when the results appear to be totally positive, there is always, for some like Beverly a trace of fear:

"The operation went beautifully, the radiation treatments were not too bad—just tiring. Drs. N. and U. said I didn't need chemo, but had the choice, which I turned down. I was able to do my housework and the cooking with little trouble; but in the back of my mind the question, would it spread? As of today it has not, the dear Lord God has been with me all the way."

And Linda P. reported doing everything in her power to prevent the return that she fears: "My biggest fear is that it will return—either in my breast or another part of my body. I changed my diet—even went to a dietician, started playing golf, go for walks with my husband and try to stay updated by reading and checking the Internet, but there are times when only a 'good cry' will do."

For others, as for Eve, the "afterward" we refer to in the chapter title includes ongoing complications:

"Dr. S. told me that after I was done with the radiation I had to take Tamoxifen for 5 years because my lump was estrogen and progesterone positive, which means that these hormones fed my cancer, and now I have to get a medicine that stops the hormone, the estrogen, from feeding the cancer cells, if any remain in my body. I took Tamoxifen for 8 months, and I felt healthy again but reality and feelings are two different situations. I felt good because

I was happy that my hair was growing back and I actually do not need more treatments just checkups, and I am a free person to enjoy life again with the hope that everything will work out for me.

"However, life is not so simple as we would like it to be. Besides my breast cancer I have a partial blockage in my right carotid, and the Tamoxifen caused a block in my left carotid too. Dr. M., Director from the Neurology took care of the carotid texts and the verdict was that the Plavix and the Tamoxifen interact and I have to decide if I want to do an internal checkup to see how bad in reality the blockage is in my left carotid. At that moment began my problems. I talked with Dr. S. who said that although I took only 8 months of the Tamoxifen I have to stop it and take the Femara—maybe it will be better for me. So he gave me Femara and I took it for 4 months, but the carotid looked the same. I tried to take Aggrenox and stop the Plavix; it was a blood thinner too with 7% aspirin in it and I am allergic to aspirin—I felt terrible. I decided to take back the Plavix to save myself from artery problems. My right carotid is stable, thank God, for 13 years, and I told Dr. S. that I will take the risk and I will not take the Tamoxifen. At that time I was not able to do more. He did not like it and told me that my cancer can come back in my other breast or in the lung. My mammogram was good and all my checkups clean, so I felt again with what I have in hope that everything will work out for me. But I am not stupid and my doctors and my family knew that I am taking high risks but it was about my life and I decided what I felt I had to do. My family supported me in everything because I had made good decisions for myself all my life. I lost my loving mom at age 15 and I had no other choices. I was praying to God to help me. I knew the risks are big and I checked my breast all the time.

"My son-in-law left Henry Ford Hospital in 2002 and I had my last checkup on 6/6/2002. Everything was normal—blood test, mammogram, cardiac examination regular—and I felt healthier when I left than when I arrived at Henry Ford. I left because I no longer had the insurance coverage.

"I would like to finish my story here, but for the fairness and real story I have to say that on 11/18/2003 I discovered a small lump in my left breast, 1.6 cm not metastatic but cancer. A completely new lump, estrogen and progesterone positive. I knew that I was at high risk because I did not take the Tamoxifen and thank God I was lucky that I do not need the chemotherapy. I was checked; CT scan, bone scan, lymph nodes, etc. Everything was OK. So my new oncologist/hematology Dr. K. decided to give me radiation therapy and Arimidex that will fight with my hormones not to create any more problems. This medicine is not blocking the arteries and I hope to feel good. I am supposed to finish my radiation in the middle of April and then I will finish my story."

Eve went on to conclude her story:

"I got my radiation therapy from Dr. L., Director, Radiation/Oncology Breast Service. She is also a very serious and good doctor and I feel lucky to be in good hands. I began my treatment on 3/1/04 and I need 31 treatments. I hope that everything will be OK but nobody can predict the future. So far so good, thank God. Today is 4/12/04 and I finished the radiation therapy. Thank God everything is OK with me I take my Arimidex and I feel healthy, and I am full of hope that this medicine is better for me. In the future I will follow my checkups mammograms and help myself with good healthy diet and exercises. I will do everything that is in my hands to be able to enjoy life because I have a passion for life. The alternative is much worse and we all will find out sooner or later what is this other world."

Despite all the setbacks, all the adjustments with medications and all the careful weighing of risks against benefits, we see that F.H. was "full of hope" and looking forward to enjoying her life. The "passion for life" that she described is a common feature of most of the breast cancer survivors who participated in this book.

These serious complications are not the rule, however. Most breast cancer survivors simply found a way to return to a version of their normal life. Joyce said:

"I followed the operation with a 5-year Tamoxifen study under the supervision of Dr. A. Tamoxifen was no problem for me. The only side effects I noticed were the first couple of years; I would have sudden hot flashes. These were so quick that by the time I noticed the flash, it was over. There were no other noticeable effects. I will complete my Tamoxifen in March 2004. I have successfully passed my mammogram and the follow-up checkups."

In a similar vein, Francine reported: "I'll be on Tamoxifen for 5 years and I experience hot flashes daily—but I'd rather have hot flashes than cancer. Since the surgery I have become a grandmother and I'm looking forward to many healthy years watching my grandson grow up."

And Yvonne celebrated: "After chemotherapy and radiation it was mostly getting my life back to normal without thinking about weekly or daily trips to the doctor's office. One day I realized I hadn't thought about breast cancer for a week. Hallelujah!!!"

Yvonne went on to note how the simple passage of time can be emotionally healing:

"Lastly, I tried to get out of bed every morning with a positive attitude and keep my lifestyle as normal as possible. And you know what, before long that one [shitty] year that nurse talked to me about was over."

Many women reported that participation in research also helped, though the tone of voice in Sharon's account is objective and matter-of-fact:

"I return each 6 months to the research department to measure my arms and mobility after the sentinel node procedure. I also had marrow removed from both hipbones and donated a vial of blood for research purposes. The hip procedure caused no discomfort, perhaps because I am so lean (5′ 5″ and 112 pounds). I lost about 3 pounds after the diagnosis because I lost my appetite, but that soon came back. I've weighed about the same since I was 18 because I've always been very physically active."

I sense how she is reassured by her own emotional and physical toughness.

Jennie balanced her return to normal life with a fatalistic humor:

"With the operation I never had any pain and 2 months later started to bowl. I do bowl now two times a week with the seniors. After my operation, because I'm on Coumadin, I was black and blue for a couple of months, but it all cleared up.

"It started in August 1990 when I had a mitral valve replaced. In September 1995 I became a diabetic, and I take insulin. In November of 2000 was my mastectomy. So I thought every 5 years I have a major health problem to look forward to! In April 2003 I had an aortic valve replaced."

The breast cancer survivors who responded to the questionnaire took the physical damage to their breasts with courage and resiliency, doing what was necessary or simply accepting what happened. Ethel noted, "Large breasts are a part of my body structure and there was some concern that there would be a noticeable change in my appearance. However, this did not happen." And Sharon said, "I've been on Tamoxifen for just over 2 years now with no side effects. My mammograms have been good since the surgery. My left breast is somewhat deflated and scarred, but nothing that is noticeable in my clothes. I don't even need a padded bra."

The "afterward" for breast cancer survivors is never as simple as resuming bowling or wearing or not wearing a padded bra. Listen to the complex mixture of feelings in what Becky said: "My niece Amy bought me blessed holy oil that I used everyday asking God to keep me alive and strong. I don't want to die from breast cancer or a car crash for that matter. Old age would be preferred. But, I accept whatever comes first. I have gone on with my life, and don't have time to cry for myself. Life is too short. When I do cry, it is for my niece Dawn, who I wish before she died would have known I shared with her this breast cancer journey."

And from Lisa: "Following surgery and radiation, Tamoxifen was prescribed, so once again I started counting, not days this time, but months, 60 in all. So far I've counted 57 so have just 3 more to go. Perhaps comfortwise, my most uncomfortable moments were those of preparation for tests, surgery, and radiation. The procedures themselves were over, in most cases, before I knew it. The little wires are gone but each time I dress or shower I'm reminded of my surgery, not by scars but several tiny blue tattoos on my right breast."

And Hardeep concluded that she suffered from "significant posttreatment depression. I did not have the treatment to focus on, as if I was not doing anything, and there might be a recurrence."

In addition to this balance of return to life against the lingering fears, many women were able to realize actual benefits from their experience with breast cancer. Listen again to what Pamela Brady said in her case study in Chapter 1: "Every time someone asks me how I am doing I get this huge smile on my face and say, 'Just fine. Thanks for asking!' and mean it. Every day is a blessing." And Beatrice who we also met earlier, combined her anger with appreciation:

"The experience is over. Visits every 6 months to the oncologists, plus the regular mammograms bring no fear. Friends have had reoccurrences of their cancer. Some survived, some did not. We live life fully each day and know how fortunate we are to be physically active. My hair is back in place and my toenails are staying intact.

"Do I have any anger? Yes—I am angry that we are living with an epidemic of breast cancer. And with all the research going on we don't know what causes it. My anger becomes hotter when young women in their 30s have to deal with this.

"I have deep appreciation for the medical community that helps each patient to feel supported and cared for. I feel particularly grateful for the warm contacts with my doctors who have been and still are there for me. Dr. D. and Dr. N. have always been most supportive . . . as have their staff."

Her appreciation includes both the medical community and her own ability "to live fully each day"—an appreciation missing in many of us who have not had cancer.

Judith also discovered an appreciation that she did not have before: "While this was a very traumatic event in my life, I learned a lot about breast cancer and have found out there are so many survivors out there that you never knew about that give you support. I was fortunate to have caught it early and more fortunate to have gone to HFHS for my treatment as their facility and the personnel are the best." She discovered she is part of a community.

Francine had a different kind of discovery: "In many ways the experience brought me closer to my husband and children. When you think about your own mortality it helps to put in perspective what is truly important in life. I am grateful for the excellent care that I received from all of the doctors, nurses, and technicians involved in this experience."

And Beverly came to a conclusion that would be almost unbelievable without all the evidence of strength, courage, and growth revealed in this book: "My father sent emails to everyone in his address book asking for prayers for me. I was on the prayer list of I don't know how many churches. I didn't doubt that I would get well. With all the improvements in the past 20 years, chemo treatments were nothing to be afraid of. I wouldn't wish this on anyone, but I wouldn't take it away from my experiences either. In fact, I think it was the best thing to happen to me in a very long time."

And Yvonne found even more positives:

"Believe it or not there are some positive to take from all this—when you lose your hair and are wearing a wig you can be ready to leave the house in just about half the time as normal. That's good, isn't it? I was 65 when I was diagnosed and decided when my hair started to grow back in to find out what color it really was under the tint. I now have silvery gray hair much like my mother had. I think she would like the way it looks.

"Another big positive are all the wonderful doctors, nurses, and support people who genuinely care about you and your returning to good health. They were a very positive force in my care and treatment, and I will always have a special place in my heart for them. I hope they all know how good they are at what they do.

"Last but certainly not least is your family—they are a tremendous source of support and love and sometimes it takes something like breast cancer to reinforce those feelings that were there all the time. Make the most of it."

I love the way her list of positives moves from the strictly practical to something much deeper emotionally.

Linda N., whom we met earlier, concluded with great insight:

"I would find it almost impossible to believe that anyone could be faced with a cancer diagnosis and not turn to his/her higher power for comfort and guidance. I will forever be grateful that *today* I am healthy. I continue to pray for the possibility of many tomorrows. I will live each day in such a way that anyone who comes in contact with me—friends or strangers—walks away with a smile. I am grateful, as odd as that sounds, for the opportunity to feel my own mortality. The world tends to be in a better perspective.

"Cancer, although a terrifying diagnosis, is not a death sentence. Medical science has given us the ability to survive this disease if it is diagnosed in the early stages. We can have the opportunity to live much better lives for having had the experience."

Her phrase, "the opportunity to feel my own mortality" is priceless. It shows the importance of *how* one sees breast cancer—or any kind of crisis. I said earlier that breast cancer survivors are remarkable for the courage and strength that they bring to the ordeal that life sent their way. Imagine what it takes to see breast cancer as "an opportunity to feel my own mortality."

Susan W. found the same fundamental courage and strength—from a variety of internal and external sources:

"After I finished my chemo my hair grew back with more body and a curl than I never had before! I was put on a drug called Tamoxifen. I was supposed to be on this for 5 years but I was switched to a drug called Evista because of uterine bleeding. Four years after chemo I had to have my uterus removed (not cancer). At this time I also opted to have breast reconstruction. I had the tram flap and was very pleased with it. Within the last year my doctor has taken me off Evista and replaced it with a drug called Femara. A new study has showed it to help prevent a recurrence.

"I am going on 6 years of being cancer free. I cherish life in a whole new light now. Not one day goes by when I don't thank God for helping me through my troubled times. He was always there to pick me up on my lowest days. Remember when you feel too weak to go on that is when he will pick you up and carry you in his arms!"

And finally, Sally Cole-Saul showed how a cancer survivor can face the future by combining efforts in her physical, mental, intellectual, spiritual, and emotional life:

"My biggest fear is that the Big 'C' might return. I try to do all the right things to keep up my immune system by sticking to organic foods and vitamins. I try to stay mentally and spiritually healthy, which helps me to deal with my fears. I feel I have a purpose on this earth and until it is completed I will continue to survive. I try to stay happy and positive. I believe that if you have all three of these things—someone to love, something to do, and something to look forward to—you generally are happy.

"We all face the unknown with uncertainty. Is there a heaven? Is there a hell? Will I get hit by a car and killed tomorrow? A cancer survivor is linked to her feelings of mortality on a real-time basis: day-to-day, month-to-month, year-to-year, test after test, sometimes hour-to-hour. I work very hard to remain an optimist. When I can maintain this outlook, I seem to acquire an abundance of resilience, which lets me deal with life's punches. Thinking positive has become my number one job in life!"

It is abundantly clear to me that Sally Cole-Saul has used her breast cancer experience as a way to discover secrets to leading a happy and fulfilling life— with or without breast cancer! She has acquired "an abundance of resilience" that many people without breast cancer can only envy.

12

Case Study—Linda D'Antonio: "A Thief in the Night"

I met Linda at a breast cancer fund-raising dinner. The uniqueness of that first conversation with Linda proved to be prophetic. I've learnt to see many hidden attributes in patients over my years of clinical practice and I can usually sum up personalities pretty quickly upon first meeting them. She was friendly, optimistic, and exuberant. She knew of me and asked me a lot of questions about myself. I'm usually the one to ask the questions; that's what doctors do. But Linda was skilled at bringing out the best in me by her quick-witted approach. We rapidly developed a rapport with each other and I knew she was passionate in her beliefs about her role in the future of breast cancer treatment and prevention. She exuded passion for supporting breast cancer research. Over the next few years I saw her at other events and became aware of her story, the subject of this chapter. Not immediately apparent is her determination to do something meaningful for others. My "Linda story" is the recognition that a determined woman can generate enough energy to raise a substantial amount of money by encouraging everyone to work hard and produce something meaningful. She made bracelets on her kitchen table, sold them, and donated a substantial sum to our breast cancer efforts. She recruited her husband and made thousands more bracelets. She had no previous experience. She just decided to do it, and she did. And she still does. Her story reminds us that compassion and tenacity are personality traits that any breast cancer survivor can strive for. Her story is unique and heartwarming.

Each of us who is a cancer survivor has our own personal story to share. Each of our stories gives personal insight into our own struggles, fears, doubts, and even hopes. While my story is not much different from many others, my personal response is truly unique.

My First Battle

It was the fall of 1990, and I was a healthy woman in my early 40s. I was married to a wonderful man, and we had four beautiful and very active children. My life was very fulfilling. I didn't drink or smoke or take drugs. When time permitted, I would exercise. My weight was good. I was always conscious of trying to live a good life.

At that time, my physician, Dr. F., was an internist. My gynecologist had retired, and I didn't see a need of a new one as I didn't foresee any problems. I had a good relationship with my internist and felt completely confident and comfortable with him. He seemed to stay on top of any health issues that needed to be addressed.

Since I was in my 40s, my doctor suggested I start having mammograms. I didn't give it much thought. After all, it was just another test; maybe a little uncomfortable but nothing that should concern me. A mammogram was just another inconvenience that I could easily fit into my hectic schedule. Cancer was never in the picture. In reality, I was too busy to even give it a thought. Cancer happens to other people, people in the papers, people in other neighborhoods. Not me.

By the time of my third mammogram, they had started to become a routine part of my visits to the doctor. But this time, a few days later, my phone rang. I found it unusual that my doctor was calling me in the middle of the afternoon. His voice was calming as he proceeded to tell me that my mammogram showed some irregularities and that he took it upon himself to schedule an appointment for me with a surgeon downtown. He said it was in my best interest to let him look over the x-rays and that he was better educated to make decisions for me. The appointment was for the following day!

I hung up the phone and tried to pretend nothing had happened, continuing with the activities surrounding me in my home. Suddenly I was confronted with something I was not sure how to digest. I just decided I wasn't going to think about what just happened. I was hoping it was just an illusion that would go away once the day ended. It didn't.

You must understand 16 years ago, breast cancer, or even the possibility of any kind of cancer, was never discussed! It was considered to be the silent killer. Automatically, someone facing cancer would be looked upon with pity. Cancer was something discussed only among family and close friends, but never with the prospective patient.

I didn't share this appointment with anyone, not even my husband. It didn't seem necessary to worry him. I think I was in a state of shock trying to fight off any fear. I concentrated on conditioning my mind to be calm and ready to accept whatever was going to happen. I was about to enter a whole new world, one I was completely unprepared for.

The surgeon, Dr. K., was marvelous. He was polite, knowledgeable, and compassionate, and he spoke to me with words I could easily understand. He took his time as he explained what he needed to do. My questions were never treated as inappropriate or trivial. For those few minutes I was with him, he made me feel that I was his only patient. He made me feel completely confident in his ability to take care of me, and I felt comfortable with his decisions. The surgery was scheduled in just a few short days.

My drive home was hazy. How was I going tell Jim, my husband, that I needed this little surgery without sounding any bit fearful? I think, at this point, the hardest part was not to prejudge the outcome. Dealing with the unknown causes our minds to make fantasy scenarios that are played as full life realities. Believe me, it's truly tough not to let our thoughts stray into this direction. I realized it was crucial that I remain in complete control. I could not at any point become emotional or weak. Those characteristics were not to be a part of the person I was about to play. But as hard as I tried, fear kept creeping in, trying to take over my body. Darn it, I was scared! How in the world was I going to disguise these emotions? Where and with whom could I share my fears?

I didn't want my children to know anything. I needed to protect them. After all, isn't that what moms do? We somehow find that inner strength to mask any fears or doubts we have. It's our job. It's our role. They would leave for school as they normally do, except this particular day they needed to know that there was the possibility I would not be there to greet them when they arrived home. I said I had to go downtown for this test and wasn't sure how long it would last.

The surgery was fine considering I woke up during the procedure to see the surgeon digging into my breast! Oops, put me back to sleep! I was numb in these strange surroundings; bright lights, all sorts of people in white! Where was I?

Recovery was, "It's finally over." I must have just been kidding myself when I thought I could handle this because immediately a massive migraine set in. Along with this migraine came bouts of vomiting. This is not a good thing! I could not be released from the hospital until the vomiting was under control. Somehow, I needed to fool everyone around me once again and try with all my might to hold back any vomiting until I was released. I just had to hurry up and get home, home secure away from anything remotely associated with this illness. Home where I knew my family was.

I know God was with me. I was able to control the vomit only to the parking lot. That was definitely good enough.

The following day I inspected my breast. It was all black and blue. It seemed strange to me to think this breast, the one that was my children's nutrition for their beginning lives, now was in deep trouble. This breast that we see all around us as a sign of womanhood was under attack. Why does society always put such emphasis on who we are by means of the way we look? How fragile and delicate our lives truly are.

My follow-up visit was scheduled in 7 days. I continued life as if nothing had happened. I pretended not to be concerned. No matter how hard I tried, every now and then thoughts would surface: Who would care for my children? Could Jim function if I wasn't around? What if it was going to be a long process of chemo and radiation? What if it was too late for anything?

I heard the news I feared the most. Dr. K. didn't use the word cancer, he just said the results were positive, but that the good news was it was caught extremely early, at the beginning stages, and that it was so small in size. He kept trying to be so reassuring as not to upset me. What he didn't know was that nothing had sunk in anyway, and I was only walking through the motions, conscientiously making sure that at no time I would be emotional and seem that I was out of control.

Then, without hesitation, words came out of his mouth that apparently back in 1990 was protocol for all patients. He offered to me three choices I had to choose from. First, I could get chemotherapy to make sure no cells had gotten away. Next, he offered a mastectomy, which would eliminate any problems of recurrence. Lastly, he said I could be closely watched to make sure nothing redeveloped. I asked which he recommended. He said closely watched and explained to me why he chose this method of treatment. I wasn't as confident as he was, but I opted to be closely watched. After all, he was the expert. Too much had already happened anyway and I just wanted to go back, back to the way my life was.

Through this whole conversation I felt as if I were up to bat in a baseball game, one fast ball after another being thrown, each with precision and each forcing me to make decisions and make them fast. I don't think I was remotely aware of what was happening.

Moments later, when my visit was over, I realized how totally uneducated I was in this area. Sure, I had heard of cancer and I knew it existed, but never, never was I the one to go to battle. I had never known anything about words like "chemo," "biopsy," or "mastectomy." I didn't even do the self-breast examinations. I was a 43-year-old woman, my life was too busy, too full, to take any precious time out for anything. But let's face it, without health, without good health, nothing else matters! I felt completely ignorant.

Like many of you, I really never paid much attention to my personal health until something happened. Then, you panic. You lose direction and nothing makes sense.

This was the start of my whirlwind journey. I could not go back to the way I once had lived. This is not possible once you realize cancer has come to visit. Whether it's a thief in the night or that uninvited guest, we must somehow learn to deal with it. It never goes away. You only hope that it behaves and with luck, remain dormant.

I had now become partners with this surgeon Dr. K., who would be my confidant, my support, and my hope in battling this disease head on. Everything happened so quickly. Looking back, I see that this was a good thing. I didn't need that extra time to ponder on what I now needed to confront head on with all my energy.

I will always be grateful to Dr. F. for his speedy care. He not only made sure I started mammograms, but he was thorough enough to follow through when it was needed. I am grateful that he scheduled that appointment quickly and then personally called me to tell me. Had any time elapsed and had he given me those responsibilities, I am sure my recovery would have been much more difficult.

This compassion is what separates a great doctor from a good doctor. To a patient, compassion matters. Dr. F. even called me after my surgery to make sure I was okay. He made himself available if I needed to talk. His reassurance gave me the comfort of knowing he cared. Doctors need always to remember that we are human beings with a name and a face, not just a patient. Treasure this gift of life that is so precious, so very precious.

I went from having mammograms every 3 months to 6 months. With the approach of each test, fear crept up and tried to overtake my body. Fear was becoming part of my new life. Faithfully, I would call to make those appointments. My relationship with the surgeon was good, and I had complete confidence in him. After each mammogram, an appointment was set with Dr. K. to discuss the results and he would reassure me of their results. How I needed that reassurance! It was like a shot of adrenaline usually getting me to the next appointment.

After approximately 2 years, my visits now were yearly. I called to make my usual appointment and was greeted with some shocking news: my surgeon had died! I froze as I listened to those words. How could this man, my doctor, my partner, who I had come to depend on for all the right answers and the right treatments—how could he die? Was it cancer? Does this cancer not care whose life it affects and when? How could this be happening? I suddenly felt deserted and alone.

I made the decision to return to my internist care. I didn't have any problems, and since my relationship with him was good, I felt confident. Once again he became my partner in health. Still, every time I had that mammogram, fearfully I would await the results. We think we are these strong human beings and we think we are prepared. We are not.

When it was once again time for my mammogram, I wasn't on top of the visit. I had let 3 months elapsed beyond my appropriate time. I was very anxious to get the results and a bit nervous that they wouldn't be okay. I called my doctors office to see what I could find out. The nurse was kind enough to look at my results and give them to me. Her voice showed grave concern; there weren't good and, "Oh my goodness! It looks like both your breasts show abnormalities!" Oh, no! Panic took over my thoughts. I cried and cried. Thankfully, it was a weekday afternoon and no one was at home. Thoughts rapidly raced through my mind. I was not in control. Did those extra months I waited cause this? Was this the verdict I was getting for not taking personal responsibility for my own health? Was this the end?

Later that day, my doctor called thinking I did not have the results. I told him what happened, and he quickly said she should have never told me that. Yes, they didn't look good, but nothing is conclusive until a biopsy is performed. His voice sounded reassuring. Another biopsy; another battle. Once again I won.

I was always on a roller coaster. The emotions ran high and low. I experienced so much anxiety followed usually by a celebration of joy. I tried hard over the years not to think about breast cancer, ignoring anything that had that name associated with it. The fear would always creep up and taunt me, and I always fought back, determined not to let it overtake my thoughts.

For the following 9 years my health was monitored closely. My personal battle to overcome the fear was more of a threat than the actual mammograms. Without any doubt, I could never have succeeded if it were not for my deep faith in God. It was God I would turn to talk about these fears. When fear threatened me, it was He who would give me the strength I needed. And when the fear became overwhelming and I was too weak, I found comfort as He would embrace me in His loving arms and carry me through whatever I was confronting. I survived each surgery in surrendering all my fears and doubts to God. He is the one who would guide my doctor in all His works. With God at my side, His presence, His love, nothing was impossible. He is the one I ultimately place all my hope in! I love God with all my heart and I cherish the extremely intimate and personal relationship we share. My God is the unconditional love, and that love is what gives me peace, peace in knowing that I am never alone.

And with that peace, I know whatever His decision was for me, I was going to be okay. I knew, too, that He was there for my family and that they, too, would be okay with whatever happened. I sometimes would feel selfish constantly asking God for His help and His protection. But I honestly can say that I could never get through life, especially battling cancer or any huge crisis, without the knowledge that my God was there with me every step and with every breath lighting the path for me to travel.

MY SECOND BATTLE

Ironically, I seldom ever talked to anyone about my feelings. I always wanted to protect my family, especially my husband. I didn't want anyone to worry about me. I was the youngest of four girls in our family. For some reason, as sisters we just never really talked about cancer. It wasn't because we didn't care about one another or didn't love one another; it was more about the way we were brought up. My parents were immigrants from Italy. Displays of love were silent. We were taught things like respect, obedience, manners, etc. There never was much discussion about anything. We knew our parents loved us, but we never saw outpourings of hugs and kisses.

My sister Rosie, who was 5 years older than me, didn't believe in the value of mammograms. Whenever we talked and I would tell her about my biopsy, she would tell me she thought I was insane. She said I would definitely get cancer from all those mammograms. I felt maybe I should just keep all these things bottled inside, so I backed off. I was the baby girl and somehow I always did things differently. They always told me I was from a different generation. I was: I am a baby boomer! We baby boomers are supposed to be changing the world. According to my sisters, I was the spoiled one. That, coupled with the fact that you really didn't share or talk about cancer, kept our discussions to a minimum.

Then the unthinkable happened. It was August 1998. I had moved and was living about an hour from Rosie. My mammogram was in February, and it was good. Besides, I had other things on my mind. I was busy planning my only daughter's wedding, and cancer now was far away. Somehow this particular day my sister, the one who didn't believe in mammograms, was on my mind. I had neglected to spend as much time as I used to with her, and I missed her. Our lives are always on the fast track; we just don't do the things that matter most. We seem to treat each day as though they never will end.

We would always do all kinds of silly and fun things. In reality, Rosie was my idol. When I was younger, I tried to imitate how she would fix her hair. She was beautiful and had a fabulous body. She would always give me her hand-me-downs, and it used to make me feel so important. It was so funny! Rosie always thought I would be the one who was destined to do great things when it was her who I admired. Her life was one of always giving to others. She spent the majority of her time raising monies to help others who were in need, especially small children. Her spirit was free, her heart filled with love and compassion. She was a really giving person.

That particular summer day she was deep in my thoughts, and I decided to drop everything and spend the day with her. I realize how often we all get so caught up in our own little worlds. I dialed her number, and I could hear fear in her voice even though she tried not to show it. She told me she couldn't spend the day with me as her doctor told her she needed a mammogram as she might have cancer. My heart stopped. I couldn't be hearing this! She broke down in tears. She was 56 years old and never had a mammogram. She had no idea of what was going on. She was scared! The pain in her breast was real. She never shared this with me. She had been in real denial. She blamed the pain on her little grandson's accidentally hitting her in the breast. Like me, she had not shared this with her husband or children or anyone. Was it her fear that kept her from taking action? Did she know deep in her heart that there was a real problem and hope that if she ignored what was happening, it would go away? Denial; why do we do that?

I quickly hung up the phone and drove to her house. It was an hour's ride. I was in a daze. I knew this was serious. I once again had to really condition myself so I could be strong for her and help her get through this. Maybe that is why I was the one who called that day.

When I arrived at her home, I found this fragile frightened woman uncontrollable and so desperate. She was completely frazzled. She quickly showed me her breast, looking for me to confirm it was nothing. I saw something I never witnessed before. It was discolored, blackened, and pitted, and I saw her nipple was inverted. I knew immediately she was in trouble. *Dear God, I need you now!* I needed to remain calm and in complete control. She didn't need me to cry. She needed a sister to give her support and to be her eyes and her ears. She needed a sister to drive her to the hospital.

After she had a series of mammograms and ultrasounds, we found ourselves in the waiting room. I watched helplessly as Rosie, paced, cried, and desperately prayed. All her fears were exposed. She did what most of us in the time of need: pray. She desperately was searching for someone to come and comfort her. Only in prayer can we find that. I couldn't change anything. I couldn't take away the fear or the pain. I only could be a support in love. I echoed her prayers in my heart.

When they gave her the results, I knew instantly it wasn't good. Rosie wasn't listening. She was so emotional that she did not have a chance to understand what was transpiring.

The prognosis was much worse than I had anticipated. It was inflammatory breast cancer, and it was advanced. The survival rate is less than 5 years if you are lucky. Along with this cancer comes pain, much pain.

What an irony. This sister, the one who warned me not to get mammograms, now was facing cancer! I couldn't believe this was happening. It was never supposed to be Rosie. It was me battling this disease for 9 years, me, who should have been the one. If I had the cancer I could deal with it. How can I help someone else? It's just like when you see your children sick and you want to take it away. When you see the one you love sick, you wish it were you. It's easier that way. You feel their pain, their anguish. How was I going to help! I wanted to control the situation. I wanted to do something!

Then came the guilt that it wasn't me dying. Maybe if I hadn't been so preoccupied with my own life, my own children, she would have had the opportunity to share the pain with me and ask me questions. If only I could have done something sooner! Maybe if I had just kept talking about cancer even when she refused to listen to me. Darn it, I was the smart baby boomer who had all the answers. What happened?

This was the beginning of a long journey for Rosie. Here was this vibrant woman who now was faced with a disease she could not control. She was like so many other women who don't place enough emphasis on their health care until it's too late. Then they look for the best doctor and the outstanding medical facility, hoping for a miracle. We pray desperately to God asking him for that miracle of life. He does hear and answers our prayers. Sometimes the answers are not what we were looking for. I don't think we will ever understand God's ways.

I was there for her as much as I could. I tried to be a sister that she could lean on. We talked, we joked, we prayed. She found peace along the way. My greatest memory throughout her ordeal was this one afternoon we were talking. She told me to make sure and take care of myself. She said she was wrong not to listen to me and that, yes, mammograms are important. She told me how sad she was that she wouldn't have the opportunity to see her grandchildren grow. But she was not at all fearful of death. She had faith that one day there would be no more pain. She was ready for her life in eternity with God. That was her real hope! As children we learned early on the importance of our faith. Rosie's pain remained, but there was the peace; peace that only God can give. He most assuredly answered her prayers. He was preparing her for her new life.

And she shared one more thing: she told me not to return to work but to spend my days helping others. She said I had the gift to impact others' lives as I had hers. She didn't realize how she was my hero! How much I had learned from her.

My Third Battle

My story doesn't end there. Suddenly I started experiencing pain in my breasts. They were extremely sensitive to touch. I thought I was just stressing over Rosie. My husband insisted I see the doctor to make sure. Feeling I was only going to bother him, I reluctantly made the appointment. I now had a new surgeon who was extremely proactive with my examination and did mammograms and ultrasounds. He was so thorough and even though the tests showed nothing, he was determined to get to the bottom of this pain. Dr. E. said he knew there had to be a problem but just couldn't pinpoint it. I could see the frustration in his eyes. Sincerity was definitely written all over his face. He told me to go home, and if the pain persisted, then I needed to return.

Six weeks later I was still having trouble so I returned. New mammograms were done. This time, three suspicious spots popped up. How could this doctor have known there was a problem? Once again, I had a great doctor.

He scheduled a biopsy. For whatever reason, I had a feeling that this was it. I just knew my choices this time around were going to be so limited. The biopsy was positive. It was like a sigh of relief. All those years fretting of the cancer returning now were coming into a reality. The emotions left me drained. Were these tests results helping me feel the burden lifted? I did not have time to concentrate on my own health, for Rosie was important not only to me, but my entire family. My mother was struggling with my sister's illness, and I was not going to burden her with this. So what plan of attack was I going to venture this time around?

Delicately, my surgeon, Dr. E., sat down with to explain in detail and on paper what had transpired. He further said this new cancer cell was caught early, but that it had invaded several areas of the breast. Therefore, I need a mastectomy. He was not only thorough but completely compassionate. Once more I felt that I was the only patient this doctor had. What happened to me mattered to him. It was his persistence that produced the early detection, and my ability to win another battle. Without him, I may not have been here to share this story.

I could no longer be ignorant of any information about breast cancer. It was my responsibility to educate myself so I could make intelligent decisions regarding my health. This was my body, and who was going to cut it had to be someone in whose ability I felt completely confident. I needed to remind myself that a doctor, as much as we would like to believe he can perform miracles, is a talented and gifted man with a license to practice medicine. So it's important to know his history, his successes, and his procedures. We have choices, so many choices. I didn't want to be another cancer statistic. I was a vital person with real fears.

Suddenly friends and acquaintances started calling, either telling me their experiences or just giving me support. It was 1999 and you could be verbal about telling others that you were in your personal battle fighting this disease. What nearly a decade had done! I decided then I was not going to be silent about cancer. I was going to share every experience I could, and I was going to stop being afraid. I was too tired, and I was too old. I was on a mission to make cancer a topic I could intelligently discuss. I was not going to die, and I wanted others to know that it was okay to talk about it. Maybe my experience could help someone. Talking about our cancer might send signals to other women and men to be aware of any changes in their bodies. Listen to what your body is saying to you! It's that gut feeling that can produce the unexpected and give you a fighting chance if there are any problems.

I read books, I went on the Internet, I made phone calls even to strangers, and sought second, third, and even fourth opinions. This miracle needed a little help from me! I asked question upon question, and some might have seemed silly, but each was delicately answered. I was getting out of the dark and I was educating myself. I knew that knowledge was power, and power ultimately gave me a choice for a competent decision about my body; power to feel completely at peace with whatever decision I made.

So now I am a survivor. It has been 6 years since I have given up my breasts. I have gone through many changes and adjustments. Unfortunately and sadly, I watched as my sister succumbed to this disease. She passed away 3 weeks after my surgery. She battled for nearly a year of pain, chemo, and more pain. Her memory and her love will always remain very close to my heart. Her words often echo as I try to fulfill her wishes.

I see and hear stories about others who battle the disease. It is so amazing to me how once you have had cancer you discover how many people's lives have been touched by this disease. Mothers, grandmothers, sisters, cousins, friends, and acquaintances: the list can go on and on. Cancer is part of our society. Cancer is that thief in the night who is so determined to take everything from us.

I remember listening nearly a year ago as newscaster Peter Jennings announced on national TV his battle with lung cancer. He told his audience that now he was joining a unique group of people who were battling this disease. No simpler statement could have been so eloquently said. He was so poised and wanted to portray the image of strength and hope.

Life does go on. Each day is so precious. I never stop counting my blessings as I watch the night turn to day. I thank God each and every morning for the opportunity to start life over again. I thank Him for opportunity to graciously accept this beautiful gift of life! I am at peace with myself. I know that there are no guarantees that cancer will not reappear. There is nothing I can do to change that. I realize that my body is only a covering of what and whom I am inside. Cancer can destroy it and torture it, but I will not let it attack my heart and my soul. My heart, my soul: that is the person I truly am.

The battle continues, and I realize it's now my responsibility to help in any way I can to do my part in fighting this disease. Every day we have new developments and new technology and someday, I hope, soon, we will have a cure.

I am a cancer survivor and I will continue on my mission to spread a message of endless love and hope.

13

ADVICE: "TRUST IN THE LORD. SEE YOUR DOCTOR"

The women who contributed to this book were generous in offering advice to others who have been diagnosed with breast cancer and to friends and family members who have become part of their treatment team. Much of that advice has emerged in the previous chapters, either directly or indirectly through the stories the women told and comments they made in the process. I think it best to simply let you hear the voices of these breast cancer survivors without any additional commentary from me.

"I have constantly reminded friends and associates of the importance of a mammogram. My advice to a friend diagnosed a few months after me, was to be comfortable with your team of medical professionals, proceed with due speed with their recommendations, and to maintain an upbeat and positive attitude.

"I have had my ups and downs—Bob reminds me of my mood swings! But I have attempted to maintain a positive attitude. I am enjoying life! I bless my wonderful medical team. I continue to follow any direction my team of physicians dictates. Cancer is a frightening disease that the medical profession is challenged to conquer. Great strides have been made—may all research efforts be successful!" (Isamay)

"My advice to women newly diagnosed with breast cancer would be to first give in to your emotions, to cry, ask why me, or whatever. When you take hold of yourself and the initial shock subsides, find a facility that has a breast cancer clinic where everyone reports to the same person or one facility, i.e., surgeons, radiation, oncology, etc. all report to HFHS. This was a frustration for me here in Kalamazoo as the surgeon was in one group, the radiation people another, and then the oncologist were under another group. There was no coordination of tests, visits, or urgency under this program and you are on your own to keep pushing for things to be done and you don't want to deal with this while you are trying to deal with the terror and unknown you are feeling when you are first diagnosed. At the clinics you will learn about all the options, and all the people involved in your care meet with you and in a group and determine what the best course of action is for you. It is very comforting to know that what is being recommended and why. Most of all pray and keep a positive outlook on things. Don't forget to laugh once in a while too. It helps to relieve the stress." (Judith)

"For all the special women that have breast cancer I can give one piece of advice: take the breast cancer as an accident that you have to go through and do your best to recover; eat well, exercise, think positive, and try to understand and know yourself. That way you will be able to do the right things for yourself. We are all human beings but we are not the same because the cause of cancer is different and our needs are different even with the same breast cancer, but good attitude helps everybody; also good diet and exercise and positive thinking. So please everybody with breast cancer try to help yourself because today we have better chances of surviving than women in the past had. I wish you success and good luck to everybody." (Eve)

"My advice to newly diagnosed breast cancer patients is to get all the information you can through reading and the Internet. The more you know the better informed and confident you will feel in your decision process." (Linda P.)

"My advice to everyone is to go and have the physical examination and checkup. Give the medics every opportunity to catch the cancer before it becomes harder to remove." (Julia)

"You *can't* change the past so look to the future. Accept help, absorb encouragement and energy from those around you. Seek a doctor and support team you have confidence in. Think not what *might* have been but what *can* be. Have faith, you too can be a *survivor!*" (Lisa)

"Trust in the Lord. See your doctor." (Bettie)

"Ask questions and research to find out. It helps lower anxiety. Talk to sympathetic individuals about your concerns. Be positive. Trust your health team. Know that *you'll recover.* My advice to others is please don't remind us cancer survivors of our illness anytime you see us. Once cancer doesn't equal always cancer." (Marianne)

"My advice to someone with newly diagnosed breast cancer: don't panic!! Go for the best help you can find. Read everything, ask questions, and enjoy the great people you meet on the road to your recovery. Many have become my good friends and feel free to talk about it." (Lucille)

"My only advice to any woman with newly diagnosed breast cancer is to find someone, preferably a woman, with whom you can discuss your feelings and concerns. I was lucky as I had my two daughters and daughters-in-law; my oldest daughter has such compassion—she is a special education teacher P.O.H.I. trained." (Beverly)

"My advice to women—period: please do not go through this alone. But do not allow anyone to nag you. Be close to God and most of all 'believe in God and in you,' have faith and have your loved ones pray for you. The power to pray is powerful. Meditate, love yourself, and think carefully what and how you can change things in your life that perhaps contribute to your illness. *Do not blame yourself*. No time for regrets, only forward. God bless you all." (Roxanne)

"I advise all newly diagnosed breast cancer patients to keep a positive attitude and to continue their normal daily activities with family, friends, and community." (Ethel)

"Take care of it immediately. Having breast cancer is a frightening ordeal. It is up to the patient to inform herself of all information about her disease. Read articles, attend lectures, compare notes with other BC patients. It is also very important to stay upbeat and have a positive attitude, *always*. Every day is an adventure—live life to its fullest." (Georgina)

"Do what doctor advises ASAP; follow orders to the letter." (Margaret)

"My advice to women with newly diagnosed breast cancer: first, learn all you can about the disease and your treatment choices so you can take an active part in decisions about your medical care; you may wish to participate in a clinical trial or a new or improved treatment; you should ask your doctor about this option if you are interested.
"Give all your fears to God in prayer.
"Maintain a positive attitude about your recovery.
"Before all else, be hopeful.
"So dare to hope; hold on to it for all it's worth." (Sonja)

"My advice to anyone in any medical situation in this day and age of great strides in medicine: don't give up, don't despair, tomorrow they may find a cure." (Jennette)

"I would say to all who have been diagnosed with cancer: Henry Ford Hospital is a place of care: (gentle, loving, care) and you can be sure they will have your interests in mind for your well-being. It was 3 years and 4 months ago I had my surgery, and I am doing great, thanks to HFH and the doctors and staff . . . and Lord, thank You, You have given me New Life Abundantly, in Jesus, Amen! Satan (stop and *calmly* think about that)." (Clara)

"The best advice I can give anyone is to make sure the doctor you choose gives you comfort and you do have faith in him. That to me is the key figure. I can't find enough praise for Henry Ford and Dr. B. The efficiency and professionalism is outstanding." (Alyce)

"Listen and learn." (Toni)

"You are not alone. There is a great medical team to give advice, help, and treatment.

"Do not despair.

"Do not hide your concerns, talk openly about everything to family, friends, colleagues at work, support groups.

"Try to think positively, do as much as possible in your daily routine.

"Pamper yourself and be good to yourself." (Heidi)

"I determined from the beginning of my treatment to make this as pleasant an experience as possible. As William James, the philosopher, said, 'People can alter their lives by altering their attitudes.'" (Elaine)

"My advice to other women is to go to HFH and don't anticipate problems. Take it day by day. It was not nearly so terrible as I thought it would be. The radiology department scared the heck out of me, telling me all the possible things that could happen, like difficulty in swallowing, necessitating a soft diet, a bad burn, shortness of breath, and possibly even breaking a rib because of damage to the bone. I cried when I heard all of this and none of it happened. Being in good health all my life and being a daily exerciser had to have helped. I wouldn't care to go through it again, but it is manageable with a good medical team and support from loved ones." (Sharon)

"My advice to women is that there are always options. It is not a death sentence, and there are always treatments available." (Hardeep)

"My advice to anyone newly diagnosed is to talk to a cancer survivor. And keep reminding yourself what incredible strides research has made and how phenomenal the treatment is today. Talk to your family and friends if they are understanding and supportive. Everyone is different—some people want to get as much information as they can, whilst others don't want any information at all, they just want to leave everything to their doctors. Feeling that you're part of your own treatment can help, even if it's just taking a look at your diet and making necessary adjustments. And don't be timid about asking for help when you need it—people really do want to help, they just don't know exactly what to do or what you need." (Susan)

"Find a breast cancer clinic that will review with you all the alternatives and guide you through the decision process for your treatment. Have genetic testing for the BRCA1 & 2 mutation. It will help you identify if you need closer follow-ups. I had it done after I had ovarian cancer, which came after two breast cancers. I have the gene mutation, which increased my chances of ovarian cancer. Additional tumor markers would have been done, and an earlier discovery of the ovarian cancer. Your children and your family need to understand their risks and options and the need to be vigilant and proactive. In conjunction with this, it is important to remain informed and up to date on your own health and health risks in general and to proactively manage your own health and your own life. No one else will do the job you can do for yourself. Keep your immune system running top notch so it can build good cells and fight off the bad ones. Don't ever forget the power of prayer.

"Remember that your mind is a powerful source of healing. Don't sweat the small stuff, think of the good stuff and laugh a lot. Whenever you have doubts about your health, tell yourself 1–100 times every day that you are disease free. Use every bit of strength and every resource you possess within. First, second, and in my case third, chances are not passed out every day. If we ignore our bodies, we may not like the direction it takes. Take each experience, good or bad, and learn from it; use your good and bad experiences to help others. Look at it as just another chapter in your book. When that chapter is complete, move on to the next chapter. Do not continue to relive the same chapter, because your book must always move forward.

"After surviving two incidents of breast cancer, ovarian cancer and a malignant brain tumor, I feel that we need another book to capture all the learning contained therein!" (Sally Cole-Saul)

14

CASE STUDY—ARLENE KALLEY: "HOPE—AGAIN"

Arlene K. and her husband are social friends of mine. She is not my patient. I didn't know the details of her breast cancer, and I did not try to access those medical details. Whenever we spent time together we would talk about the things that friends usually talk about. One evening we were eating dinner at a restaurant and my curiosity got the better of me. I mentioned that I had a patient who asked my advice about what to tell her teenage daughters. There is a myriad of possible responses, and the most honest is that it depends on the psychodynamics of the family. I asked Arlene what she had shared with her 17-year-old daughter who was born about 5 years after her treatment. She had told her nothing.

When Arlene was diagnosed with a recurrence over 20 years after the initial treatment, her husband called to ask my advice. Arlene had surgery at a nearby hospital, did well and came home. Imagine my amazement when, a few weeks later, she was interviewed about her breast cancer for the local evening TV news! This was the same person who previously confided in me that she was a private person and hadn't shared her diagnosis with her daughter. Now she was sharing her diagnosis with everyone. Her daughter now also knows, of course, and Arlene is a lot more forthcoming about her disease with me. Her approach to managing her experiences, emotions and feelings has been based on her ability to look at herself realistically.

I thought her experiences remarkable, and her wise approach to her disease worthy of this book, even though the rest of the book focuses on patients who have had their breast cancers treated relatively recently and have not, in general, had major recurrences. My intention was not to compile a book relating the experiences of patients with advanced breast cancer but to concentrate on early breast cancer and to expose feelings and emotions at each step of their management. The psychological aspects of more advanced cancers are discussed in other publications. However, emerging from her story are the common themes of strength, tenacity, humor, and hope. In contrast to the stories of other patients in this book, Arlene has been down the first road, and showed that, despite her devastating loss of a breast as a young woman, she was able to recover, marry, have a child, and lead a happy, productive life for many years.

Arlene's description gives her experiences first hand:

Our memories are complicated, slippery things; memories that we thought were long buried have a way of clawing them back up to the surface and events and emotions that we were sure were indelible can become faded and transformed with the passage of time. My confrontation with cancer began a quarter of a century ago; the memories of the early times are distilled down to those that are most intense. As every cancer patient knows, hearing those three words "you have cancer" from the doctor changes her life forever. My moment came in the recovery room after a biopsy on a lump I had discovered myself. My surgeon put one hand on my shoulder and with the other, tweaked my ear affectionately; he whispered that I had breast cancer. Even through the haze of the fading anesthetic I knew it was an important moment, and it stays with me to this day. My personal battle had begun. As one member of my support staff put it, I was in the ring for round 1.

ROUND 1

After the mastectomy, I stayed in the hospital for several days; I remember little of it except for the first time I took a bath without dressings. I looked at myself, deformed and mutilated, a feeling that would be permanent. In those days, a patient had to wait 6 months before getting an implant, so the shock of the removal of a breast was great. I was only 35 years old, unmarried and childless. Chemotherapy began and so did another loss to my vanity; my hair started to fall out. My hairdresser ordered a wig for me, but before it arrived she braided my hair in tiny braids all over my head to try to keep what remained in place. A few days later, I awoke in the middle of the night with a violently itching scalp. I decided to take action. After getting a brown paper grocery bag and a large glass of Scotch, I stood in front of the bathroom mirror. Little by little I took out the braids and put the hair in the bag. By the time the Scotch and the hair were both finished, I saw in the mirror a reflection that was both me and not me; a bald woman. I took the bag of hair, and with a scarf over my head, silently crept out into the hall of my apartment building and put the bag down the incinerator chute.

Is there any point in rehashing the vomiting, the fatigue, the bruises from the IVs, the determination to lead as normal a life as possible? Does time actually slow down during these events? My surgeon had a massive stroke and died; he was only in his 50s. Changing doctors was disruptive and sad.

I was teaching, but it became impossible; I went on disability. As soon as I could, though, I had surgery to put in a silicone implant; one baby step toward healing. During my second year of chemotherapy, my mother was treated for uterine cancer; my father was beside himself. He said that if my mother died he would kill himself; it was not an idle remark. Emotions were large and rampant. I had a team of supporters that was truly remarkable, comprised of my new doctor, an oncologist, an oncology nurse, a social worker, and Joann, the department secretary who coined the boxing analogy and kept all of us organized. Except for a certain few events, that whole time is a blur. I can smile now at one terrible day:

My real human hair wig was at the salon getting "done" and I was wearing an inexpensive synthetic one from the department store. I opened the oven door to check something that was baking and felt the top of the wig get weird. It had fizzled, melted, and then fused together in a molten lump. I had to get another one right away, but how could I go to the mall? I put the wig on backward and a scarf over the top; it didn't fit very well but it would do. One block from the mall I stopped for a traffic light and felt a huge "boom"; I had been "rear-ended". My first reaction was to look in the mirror; of course the ill-fitted backward wig and scarf getup had slid sideways. I fixed it the best I could before meeting with the other driver to settle our fender-bender and then purchased a new wig as quickly as I could. All I could think about was that if I had been hurt and gone to the hospital what they would have thought of my demented headgear!

Less than a month after the end of the chemo, I threw my wigs into the garbage, enjoying my newly grown fuzz. I felt I had won round 1. I dutifully reported to the hospital on a regular basis for tests, and was followed closely.

The ensuing years brought many ups and downs. Four years after my surgery, I was married and 2 years later gave birth to my daughter after a normal pregnancy. I remember so clearly showing up at the hospital to announce my pregnancy and having the doctor sweep me up in a bear hug and swing me around. They were all so proud of me and of themselves. I brought baby pictures every time I went for a checkup and Joann displayed them on a file cabinet with magnets. They referred to my daughter as "our baby." It must be remembered that it wasn't common back then to have a baby past 40, even for a "healthy" woman. It wasn't long after this that both Joann and my oncologist died, she of, ironically, breast cancer, and he of a heart attack. They were both under 50. We were devastated, but the worst was yet to come. My very closest friend was my first cousin; we were only a few months apart in age and had shared some of life's great moments. When she called me to tell me she had liver cancer, it sent me into a real tailspin. She lived for 17 more months, and as I sat at her bedside the day she died, I cursed cancer in all its forms. She was only 42 and left behind a son and a 3-year-old little girl. Not even my own illness caused me to weep as much as her passing did.

How do we get the strength to soldier on? Probably because we carry with us, up until that final moment, the ability to hope for the best. I spent the next 15 years buoyed up by my husband and by the raising of my child. During those years my father had prostate cancer and my mother breast cancer. We were beginning to think we were cursed, but also that we were survivors.

ROUND 2

Two years ago, my doctor suggested that it was time for me to get a routine colonoscopy; I opted for a "virtual" one. In retrospect it was a lucky decision. The virtual scan also shows the entire abdomen. Two days later my doctor called me on my cell phone and requested that I get to her office ASAP. "We need to talk", she said in a shaky voice. The colonoscopy scan showed two ominous things; there were bright areas on my pelvic bones and fluid surrounding my lung. Entering into my life now was a new oncologist. Right behind him came an orthopedic oncologist and a thoracic surgeon. I had a new team. The first biopsy was on my bones; a half dozen samples were taken in the hospital and declared to be arthritis. The second time, a tube was inserted through my back and more than a liter of fluid drawn out. A few days later I received a phone call telling me that the fluid contained cancer cells—*breast cancer cells*. I was stunned. How could cancer have escaped the kind of heavy-duty chemo I had? Where were the cells hiding for 20 years? I pictured a small group of nasty little delinquents rushing around trying to evade a tidal wave of poisonous chemo for 2 years and finding a safe haven in the lining of my lung, dormant until it was safe to rear their ugly heads once again and continue reproducing.

In the years since my first treatment, new drugs have appeared. One of those is the Aromatase inhibitor; over the course of the next few months, the rest of the fluid on my lung disappeared, or at least became undetectable by chest x-ray. I could breathe better and worked all that summer on my fitness and my tennis game. I only knew that I had to live to see my daughter, then a junior in high school, through to adulthood. By the time a year had passed, I was feeling great, except for the side effects of fatigue and joint pain. I am willing to put up with them to keep the cancer at bay. I had won round 2.

ROUND 3

By an eerie coincidence, exactly 1 year ago today, January 4, 2005, I had a routine mammogram on my remaining breast. The following day the radiologist called to get me back to the hospital for a digital mammogram. It showed a lima bean-sized lump deep in my right breast. A needle biopsy the next week proved it to be a malignancy, *but not the same kind of cancer as the others!*

This was a new, totally discrete event, not a metastasis. I couldn't believe it. Into my life now came a new member of the team, a surgeon. I opted for another mastectomy, figuring that at least I would match on both sides! If I had just the lump removed, I would have to go through radiation; being treated for two different cancers at the same time seemed like too much. In February I had a mastectomy, and not only was my implant put in at the time by my plastic surgeon, but also I was home from the hospital the same day. Things have changed! With a small device pumping a local anesthetic to the surgery site for the first day or so, I needed only over-the-counter painkillers for a few days, and spent a few more wallowing in bed with my Valentine's Day Godiva chocolates. Ten days later I was featured on a television news special about outpatient mastectomies. I believe I have won round 3. At this point, I would like to abandon the boxing analogy and pick up a baseball one—three strikes and the cancer is *out!*

What does the future hold? None of us knows. My father recently succumbed to the long-time spread of his cancer. He was 91. My mother, nearly 92, is healthy. Among the three of us we have had seven cancer occurrences. I am not a spiritual or philosophical person by nature, but rather a bit of a cynic. I really do not believe there is some sadist supernatural being sending cancer cells to people to kill them slowly or to see how they react. Instead I assume a certain randomness, or an inability of my body to repulse these renegade cells that surely must live in all of us. I lived to see my daughter graduate last June and go off to college; my legacy to her is twofold. While she may very well inherit the possibility of breast cancer, I hope she also inherits my stamina and optimism. Of course I have my sleepless nights, wandering around my house shaking from anxiety, but also sunny days when I plan a trip to Spain with my husband to celebrate my sixtieth birthday this fall. I would say to her, or any woman, to keep her chin up, her wig straight, fight for her life, and never misplace her strongest weapon—*hope.*

15

CASE STUDY—WILLIAM C. RANDS, III: "YOU HAD A MASTECTOMY?"

There are a number of unique insights in this chapter. Did you know that men get breast cancer? For every 100 women with the disease there is 1 man with breast cancer. Bill didn't know even when he found a lump in his breast. He didn't worry about it, thinking it was something benign. Nothing in his experience alerted him to the possibility that this could be malignant. In contrast, every woman with a breast lump knows that it could be cancer.

When he was given the diagnosis, Bill used his considerable intelligence to research the data. He came to me armed with information. I love patients who are curious, inquisitive, and want the best treatment possible. I love the challenge that Bill brought from his perspective as a new patient whose expertise is in business, banking, and investments. I felt an instant understanding while answering his thoughtful questions. He wanted details and I gave him everything I knew. He seemed to have exhausted all the questions and we set him up for surgery. But he called again the next day and I knew we had to meet face to face a second time because he had uncovered more questions that could not be adequately addressed on the telephone.

In the middle and late 1990s we were doing studies on sentinel node biopsy in breast cancer. Clinical trials were conducted throughout the country and we were the first in Michigan to offer this new technique on an experimental basis. Surgeons who wished to introduce this new technique could only do so under the umbrella of a protocol approved by the Internal Review Board. The consent process for sentinel node biopsy did not include men, and I purposely avoided discussing this topic with Bill and offered him instead the standard operation: a complete axillary lymph node dissection. When we discussed this topic at our second meeting he had become aware of sentinel node biopsy and naturally wanted to explore the possibility of having this procedure himself. He is a person of considerable intellect and logic, and we finally came to a "meeting of the minds": I agreed to do the sentinel node biopsy on him with the express understanding that we would do it "off protocol." I spent a lot of time telling him all the reasons why the new technique was experimental and why I couldn't vouch for its accuracy.

His sentinel lymph node showed evidence of tumor spread, and he carefully describes this in his story. The current recommendation is to remove the rest of the lymph nodes in the armpit, but Bill declined to undergo a second operation. I was quite disturbed by this approach, but I accepted his wishes. I'm a strong believer that people have instincts about their treatment and don't respond well to doctors ordering them around. He describes his management in the chapter. Even now, 7 years later, we still do a second operation when the sentinel node is positive, although much data has accrued and many surgeons are now of the opinion that some patients may not need the second procedure.

His story focuses appropriately on his own experiences with breast cancer. He is a humble person and a supporter of many philanthropic causes in Detroit, but he doesn't include that in his story here. He and his wife, Happy, have endowed a chair in Breast Cancer Research, which will greatly benefit present and future generations of breast cancer patients. This book describes the many wonderful stories I've been privileged to share with my patients; they have taught me how to be a better physician. Bill taught me that I can be a friend to my patients.

Here is his story:

I consider myself incredibly fortunate. Like most men, I didn't even know that I could get breast cancer. But it developed in a place where it could be removed, I was lucky enough to find it early, and I had great medical care and support. I would not trade what I have learned and experienced in this journey for anything, and in that sense I would have to say it has enriched my life more than it has impoverished it. In deference to the many, many people whose journey is much tougher than mine, I must state that I would not utter that previous sentence if I did not feel I could consider myself a survivor. I have lived to go on to other things and to do my tiny bit to help others and to fight the tragic and burdensome disease of breast cancer.

If I could offer two pieces of advice to anyone who finds herself, or importantly himself, on such a journey, these would be the following. First, there are times when you will just go along with what the doctors say, because there is no logical choice. But there are also times when there are real choices and if you are ready to take control of your care when the time is right, it will help you a lot, both physically and emotionally. Second, we cancer patients and survivors really stick together. The support and advice I received from fellow patients (of course mostly women) has been overwhelming and absolutely vital to my outcome. A consequence of this thought is that we each have a duty to help others when we can. What seems like a piece of mundane factual information from someone who has been through it can be a wondrous lifting of the fear of the unknown. I have felt comfortable being completely open and communicative about what I have experienced. Actually, when I started writing this, I worried that it would be a bad experience to relive a part of my life that was really difficult at the time. But it has been very positive for me, and I hope the result is not too colored by the happy outcome to be useful to the reader.

The communications that I have had with people about their breast cancer and mine have taken forms that range from the heartrending to the bizarre. One long-time woman friend started her chemo, for ovarian cancer, at the same time I did. We supported each other and traded many ideas about what to do, where to find information, and who to consult. I remember visiting her in the hospital when her husband was coming with their daughter to celebrate the daughter's birthday. I arrived a few minutes early and she said, "Come on, we're taking a walk." She wanted me to help her walk around the building, pushing her IV carrier. That was a tough one for me because she died a few months later, and I had to learn a little about survivor's guilt. Another woman I was asked to visit welcomed me into her living room.

"You had a mastectomy?"

"Yes," I said.

"Can I *see* it?"

I had been in her living room for 30 seconds and I had my shirt off! I was actually able to refer her to Dr. Nathanson and save her from a double mastectomy. A group of men I work with in boat racing said, "Don't say breast cancer, that's not manly. Say you have chest cancer." I replied that I would much rather have breast cancer because you can get rid of that! And being identified with a bunch of heroic women didn't bother me at all.

I discovered it in the shower. I couldn't figure out why a spot right next to my right nipple seemed hard and somewhat sore. It was August 1999, at our summer cottage, which is on Lake Huron and not near to my doctor's office. I didn't know what it was, but I knew it was something I didn't understand and didn't like. I was about due for an annual physical, and so a week later when we were home I made an appointment. I loved my doctor, a guy who would talk to me as an intellectual colleague and not a patient to be ordered around. Sadly, soon after that, he died of kidney cancer himself. We had jousted a bit about whether I would accept the idea of taking a blood pressure medicine. He never talked down to me; he just presented me with the medical evidence. Also he had said I would benefit from losing a few pounds.

I remember the physical examination very well. I actually had it in my mind to notice whether he would find the lump, and he did not. But when he was finished he said, "Now, is there anything else you would like to talk about?"

I said, "Here, check this out."

He felt the lump and said, "Well, I see about three of these a year in men, but I have yet to find the elusive male breast cancer. However, I definitely want to get this biopsied."

He made an appointment for me with the plastic surgeon in the same clinic, and about a week later I was in his office. It seemed a little weird that he took a picture of my chest before he started the biopsy, so I absorbed myself in admiring the closeup lens on the camera because it had little light sources right around the lens. He numbed the area but I remember that when he went back for some more tissue he went beyond the margin of the anesthetic. Ouch! He made some comment about the biopsy not leaving much of a scar but if it turned out to be cancer it would require some "disfiguring surgery." I recall that remark not being very reassuring at the time, but I rested my emotions on my doctor's comment that he did not expect it to be anything significant. I had to wait a week for the results.

One week later was the morning of my fifty-sixth birthday. It was 8 o'clock in the morning and I was sitting on the plastic surgeon's examining table with my legs hanging over the side. He approached me with a piece of paper, and said, "The report is positive for carcinoma." All the blood went out of my head. I really had to hold on to the table to keep from falling off. The doctor gave me the one-page pathology report and I read: "Carcinoma of the breast, poorly differentiated, grade 3." I remember asking him what the grade meant and he said that the cancer was aggressive. After I composed myself and was told I would have an appointment made for me with a doctor named N., I took the one-page report to my own doctor's office in the Internal Medicine Department.

I asked them to make a copy of it for me and to give me an envelope. I wrote on the report, "Gary, you found it this time," and left it for my doctor. I went home to tell my wife and we cried together. We called our daughter in New York and she cried with us. We called our son in Colorado, who was quiet and stunned. Later that evening my doctor called me at home. He said, "Bill, what happened?"

"Well, you told me you wanted me to lose a few pounds."

"Yes," he said, "but not this way!"

I said something about the blood pressure medicine, and he said, "Let's not worry about that right now."

Doctor N. is an impressively neat and efficient man with a kind, calming disposition and what I thought at first was an Australian accent but which I later learned is South African. I could tell he was a special doctor by the relationship he had with his staff, especially the nurses. After examining me briefly and looking at the pathology report, he rolled his chair toward me and said, "You need a mastectomy."

Huh? I couldn't even translate the word in my mind. But there seemed no turning back. Dr. N. explained that it would be outpatient surgery and that we needed to do it quickly because he was going out of town for an extended conference and did not want to wait until he would return. He asked me a few questions aimed at finding out if there was any gross spreading of the cancer, and I remember he asked me if anything hurt. I blurted out, "My foot hurts."

He said, with a little smile, that it was unusual for breast cancer to spread to a person's foot. He then said, "I'm going to ask you to do something funny; I'm going to ask you to go downstairs and have a mammogram."

I actually did not find it difficult, and now when women complain about them I say, "Well, my mammogram wasn't that bad."

During my first two visits with Dr. N. I learned something that now seems quite obvious to me: when I am in a doctor's office and being told something that will change my life forever I lose track of all the questions I was going to ask, and when I come out I can't really remember what happened. So I have taken to writing notes on a little piece of paper. I think I remember most of what went on during the first visit, but I know that during my second appointment, when he was explaining that there was about a 30 percent chance of lymph node involvement, I mostly went blank. When I got home all I knew was that I had to go in for surgery and that the surgery itself would reveal more bad or good news that I would have to deal with.

Shortly after that visit when there was less than a week to go before the surgery, a most important thing happened. I began to learn how important we cancer patients/survivors are to each other. I was talking on the phone with an old friend who had just finished her chemo and radiation, and she said, "You must ask about Sentinel Node Biopsy. I didn't have it but I wish I had." This simple statement started me on a path of learning and questioning. I learned that Sentinel Lymph Node Biopsy, or SLNB, was an ancillary surgical procedure aimed at avoiding the removal of 25 or so lymph nodes around the underarm and breast area, which had a complication rate of 50–60 percent. The complications are ugly: weakness, pain, swelling of the arm, loss of motion, all of which would have impacted me greatly because I lead an active life.

I asked Dr. N. about SLNB the next day. He said, "Yes, I did not mention it to you because I did not know how interested you would be, but we are one of the pioneer groups in the country developing Sentinel Node Biopsy." He very patiently answered a number of questions for me and for my wife and then emphasized that I had to make a decision in about 24 hours because he had to get the team together, and my surgery was scheduled later that week. Now the responsibility was really on me.

This was the first of several times when I had to prepare myself to make a decision. Off to the Internet I went and found one of the original studies on SLNB, headed by a Dr. Krag. The article stated that the procedure was new and the outcomes were heavily influenced by the proficiency and degree of synergy of the team performing it. The error rate was quoted at about 4 percent, and Dr. N. later said that in 300 surgeries his team had established an error rate of 2.5 percent. I took an older friend—who had been a mentor to me and many of my friends—to lunch and ran through the logic with him: I had to trade a potential 2.5 percent greater chance of missing lymph node involvement for the avoidance of what I felt was almost certain permanent loss of function. I chose SLNB.

The day of surgery came so quickly; it was dizzying. Talking about it gives me the opportunity to tell about my wife and how she supported me through this whole journey. Her name is Elizabeth, but she is called Happy, and she really deserves to have been mentioned earlier because she is so strong and has so much common sense, medical and otherwise. She even subscribes to two medical journals! We arrived at the hospital so early it was still dark, and she was with me during the first part of the procedure in Nuclear Medicine. This involved the injection of a radioactive tracer at the tumor site, which was tracked on a detector screen to find the "sentinel" lymph node.

When she saw the lymph node light up on the speckled screen, Happy said, "It looks like a star appearing in the night sky!" After the doctor found the Sentinel Node—and marked it with a Sharpie pen—we proceeded to pre-op. I remember being told, "You'll have to wait a while, because Dr. N. is taking longer with the patient before you." I was in an upbeat mood, bolstered, no doubt by sedatives. I said, "That's fine. I know that when it is my turn he will do the best he can do for me, too." I had heard that he drives OR teams nuts with his insistence on perfection in his surgery. I actually was happy for a few more minutes in pre-op, because a dear friend of mine, who was in much worse trouble, was there at the same time, and we could talk over the screen between our gurneys. He died 4 months later.

The next thing I remember was that I was on my way home, with Happy driving, in the dark of the evening. With the pain meds I really felt pretty good, and I was very thankful that I didn't have to stay in the hospital. The most salient feature of my chest at that time was a large bandage covering a drainage tube with a reservoir attached to the end of it. We had been taught a fairly complex procedure, which included measuring the amount of drainage and keeping track of it, and then disposing of it without triggering an infection. I remember a definite instruction not to wash out the reservoir, or, it said in very large type, I would have a "VERY BIG INFECTION." That was enough to convince both of us to be extremely careful, and Happy did a superb job caring for the drainage apparatus!

The next few days were somewhat of a blur, but pretty soon I was back in Dr. N.'s office with Happy receiving the news that one of the lymph nodes did have some cancer involvement. The magic number was 3, however, and I had less than three nodes involved. In that sense the news was good, but the doctors definitely wanted me to have chemotherapy. The other thing that stood out about that visit was the removal of the drainage tube by one of Dr. N.'s colleagues. It was like a giant worm, much longer than I had realized, and it just came out and came out and came out. It was only mildly uncomfortable, but a very strange feeling indeed.

At this point in my journey I started to learn the elements of a tumor's dossier, and particularly mine. How big was it? Two and a half centimeters. Was it positive for responsiveness to estrogen and progesterone? Yes. Was it positive for overexpression of the HER2 marker? That was a complicated one. I was told 2+ on a scale of 3. I will say more about that later. I learned that men get breast cancer about one one-hundredth as often as women, and in general are not offered nearly enough education about it. But my road would follow the same path as a woman's, with all the same fears and struggles. A man does have the benefit of two exceptions to this equality: I did not feel that my body image was threatened in the same way as a woman's by the loss of a breast, and my loss of hair, which was never complete, was an annoyance but not a source of any great embarrassment. I mention the things I learned about my cancer not because anyone needs to memorize them or because I particularly understood them, but this has become a new language for me, and when I talk with a fellow cancer patient I always start by asking these nitty-gritty questions. This approach takes a bit of the fear away for me and it seems for many other people. The point is, we can do something about cancer, and there is more information all the time that helps doctors know what to do.

This was also the point in my journey when I received the news about what I should do for chemotherapy. My oncologist sent me for a number of tests, among which was something called a MUGA, which stands for some fancy words that relate to the ability of your heart to tolerate the rigors of chemotherapy. He said that mine was not bad but not on the strong side. That statement made me feel somewhat inadequate, because it seemed to mean that I was not able to undertake the very strongest treatment. But he recommended a somewhat "milder" cocktail given over nine treatments instead of the stronger mixture for four treatments. He reassured me that it was the "gold standard," and would have an equal beneficial effect. But it did mean that I would be on chemotherapy for about 7 months. And he was anxious to start right away.

A small extra bit of surgery that people should know about was the insertion of a MediPort. This is a device under the skin of either the chest or the arm—mine was in my chest on the side opposite the mastectomy—which allows the chemotherapy to be administered without always having to find a peripheral vein in which to insert the IV. Especially for people having the stronger forms of chemotherapy this is a very desirable strategy because the chemicals can be irritating to the veins. For me it made it much easier to have chemo and much less painful.

An oncology office that conducts an active chemotherapy practice is a busy place. The one I went to was a private physicians' group that routinely did chemo for the Henry Ford System's patients on the East side of Detroit. It had a finely organized hum of activity that at first intimidated me. There were the people to weigh you and take your blood sample and get you ready to see the doctor before chemo, the nurses who administered your chemo, and then the administrative ladies who sent you away with a lollipop and appointments for any tests that the doctor wanted done. I had always had a collegial relationship with the doctors, but nurses could be very authoritative, in a kind way, of course. I was to take certain drugs the 2 days before chemo, and then report back in 5 or 6 days for a set of blood tests. What I eventually found was that the whole routine represented accumulated wisdom, most of which fit me fine, but I ran into some things that I was to challenge.

One of the drugs in my chemo mix was notorious for causing sores in the mouth, and I was taught a technique of holding ice water in my mouth when that drug was administered. It is called hydrotherapy, and the rule was you had to keep ice water in your mouth for 45 minutes. This was just to keep the blood vessels in my mouth constricted, not for the purpose of swallowing any of the water. What I am talking about here should not be confused with hydration, which is a necessary routine to keep the body supplied with water by drinking at least eight glasses a day. I was instructed that hydration is important for carrying away the products of the chemo, and works very well.

I don't know why but I really disliked the ice water trick. I got to the point that doing it during chemo actually nauseated me. Even the sound of ice clinking in a glass caused a negative reaction, and just writing this I can feel the revulsion for the ice water over that period of time. It was a small thing but they kept insisting on 45 minutes, but that last 15 minutes was just hell. Between chemo sessions I dived into the Internet and found a clinical study in which patients had used hydrotherapy for 30 minutes and 45 minutes, and 30 minutes worked just as well. I marched in with a printout of the study and announced that I was only going to gag for 30 minutes and not 45. My chemo nurse said, "Mr. Rands, why do I not put it past you to find a clinical trial to prove your point?" From then on it was 30 minutes.

I laugh at this in hindsight because I could have refused the ice water altogether, obviously at my own risk. But those people were taking care of me, and I never thought of refusing, only of minimizing the part I did not like. And the nurse's reaction was so uplifting to me: with a sense of humor and even a bit of admiration she acknowledged the validity of my logic, without giving up her authority to stick to the necessary parts of the protocol. In fun my oncologist and some of the nurses started calling me "Dr. Rands."

It was right around this juncture when I asked my oncologist if he could refer me to someone he trusted for counseling. He gave me a referral that turned out to be very satisfying, a psychologist who really understood the issues patients face: the discontinuity and the threat to one's sense of identity that cancer represents. But I think the counseling also helped me to understand the way this experience could strengthen me as a person and make me appreciate the value of life, no matter how long or how short. It also underscored the importance of the relationships and the opportunity to help people and be helped by people. It reinforced the nobility of one's actions in coping with the cancer and the ordinary challenges of life.

The balance between going along with professional advice and making my own decisions became more serious when I started using Neupogen. This is truly a wonder drug, but very expensive, which was luckily not an issue due to our excellent health insurance. Chemotherapy kills cancer cells, but it also kills a portion of the white cells in your blood, which are the infection fighters. My normal white cell count of around 3,000 went down to 1,000 or so 5 to 7 days after chemotherapy, low enough that I was relatively helpless against all the normal bugs that float around. I had to postpone one of my chemo sessions because my counts were too low, so I, like so many people before me, really needed help to recover from the depressing effects on my blood chemistry. Neupogen is a miraculous biotechnology drug that "gooses" up the white count, and this drug really works! It comes in small vials and is administered once a day under the skin with a hypodermic needle, for a period of days following the chemo infusion. The oncology office routinely told me to take ten shots.

When I came in for a blood test my white count would be 30,000+, so I began refusing to take ten shots. After each chemo I took five and it worked just fine, with my count up to 5,000 or 6,000. I had to fight a bit for that piece of autonomy, but I finally prevailed.

On the lighter side, the nurses taught me how to give myself the shots, and I remember with great warmth that one was kind enough to come to our house to coach me. I do have a moderate amount of padding around my middle to use as a target. It takes some training if you have never given yourself a shot, but it really beats going to the office every day. One wonderful detail is to use one needle to fill the syringe and then to put on a new one, so that you get a painless shot with a really sharp needle. I remember coming to a moment in the office when I needed a Neupogen shot and taking the syringe from the nurse, I said, "I'll do that." It was not a nurse I knew well, and she looked at me oddly but gave it to me and then helped me confirm that I had learned to give myself the shot properly.

When I went in for each chemo session Happy was always with me. I had my CD player and a book, usually about science because I love studying science and somehow it soothed me. The office had big overstuffed chairs and blankets, so physically it was quite comfortable. But it also had a lot of people who were quite unhappy or at least did not want to be there. Sometimes we made friends and supported each other, and sometimes people just wanted to be alone. Happy said we lived for a while in two worlds. We lived with the cancer but tried most of the time to integrate it into our regular world, but every 3 weeks we found ourselves face to face with the real world of cancer, which was like an isolated island we had to visit for a few hours.

I was blessed that I did not have much stomach reaction from the chemo. We were delighted when the much feared nausea and vomiting did not happen. Despite the preventive treatments that are available, I was conscious that many of my fellow patients suffered greatly from the stomach effects of chemo, and not having them made a big difference to me. I lost a lot of hair but kept just enough so that people would not look at me and notice a big change. I developed a format I called Bill's Daily Chemo Sheet, which helped me keep track of everything from my temperature and diet to my bowel status, so that I could give a full report when I went to the office and the doctor or the nurses had questions. I really did not miss much work except for the day after the first few chemo treatments and the one bad reaction I mentioned earlier, which happened before I started using Neupogen. So other than taking precautions against catching infections, life went along pretty well. I asked some friends at our local hospital to give me some bottles of the antibacterial cleaner they dispense for washing hands. We kept it around the house until Happy and I realized that it smelled really bad in the confined space of our bathroom at home.

One challenge that shook me greatly was caused by a friendly gesture from a close associate. He had some contacts at another cancer institute nearby, and wanted me to get a second opinion about my chemotherapy. I actually talked to one of the doctors, who said my chemo regime was all wrong and I should have a much higher "dose intensity." He actually gave me some copies of scholarly papers on the subject, and I read them carefully. In the end, I decided to stick with the people I trusted.

I promised I would say more about the HER2 issue. This is about a cellular growth gene called HER2/neu that, when it is overexpressed, indicates that the cancer is very aggressive and needs to be dealt with differently. As a consequence of my 2+ evaluation the oncologist recommended four more treatments with a different drug, so I actually had thirteen chemo treatments. Those last four treatments were really tough. I was told that some people had an immediate severe reaction to the drug, which would happen during the first few minutes of the first infusion. I really was scared. We waited anxiously, but fortunately it did not happen. I usually stayed home in bed for a day with achy flu-like symptoms after each treatment. It also made my hair fall out faster, and with each infusion my fingernails and toenails stopped growing for a day. After four treatments there were four little transverse creases in each fingernail and toenail at intervals of a half-millimeter or so, which I took to be the equivalent of the 3-week interval between treatments. In about 4 months they grew out to the ends of my nails and were gone.

The last chemo treatment, in August of 2000, was a real occasion for celebration. The nurses all congratulated me, and I felt very good. They gave me a wonderful T-shirt with an inscription that said, "It's over!!" and a picture of a fat lady singing. Ironically, we had driven 2 hours down from our cottage, which was where it all began with that discovery in the shower, and then drove back afterward. Our daughter and her friends had festooned the cottage with balloons and "congratulations" signs. It was a wonderful day!

Another consequence of the report from the HER/2 test was that the usual follow-up treatment with Tamoxifen was not recommended because of the "positive" HER2. But in fact the test that I had for HER2 turned out to be obsolescent and in the process of being replaced by something called a FISH test. After my chemo was completed I requested a FISH test and it came back negative for HER2 overexpression! At first the mix-up bothered me, but about that time my oncologist retired and the oncologist that succeeded him on my case reassured me that I was much better off because of the extra chemo treatments. He also recommended another drug called Arimidex instead of Tamoxifen because follow-up treatment has been shown to be very beneficial.

All during my chemotherapy, which because of the extra four treatments took the better part of a year, I was concerned about whether I was going to get a recommendation for a course of radiation. I did not want it, but I did not feel that this was something I could refuse if it came along. I did, however, do as much research as I could. What I found was that in general I would not be a candidate for radiation because I had had a modified radical mastectomy, meaning that the delicate question of margins around the tumor had been removed.

There was one qualification to that good news, however. If the tumor were of a type that "crumbles" and leaves the area around it and any involved lymph nodes strewn with dangerous crumbs of tumor, radiation would be appropriate. I went into my appointment with the radiation oncologist thinking that I was going to say something very wise and philosophical, like, "Well, I am happy not to have radiation but that's good and bad news, because you are saying to me that this isn't a tool that will reduce my chances of a recurrence." Harrumph harrumph. When the time came to hear the words and she said that she was not going to recommend radiation, I was so happy that all I did was burst into tears!

It was in the late fall of 2000, just about a year after I found that lump in the shower, when my journey of being a patient gave way, in my mind at least, to a journey of survivorship. I was still on a pretty short leash, with checkups every 6 months and then finally every year. At first each checkup was a threat. What if the cancer came back? I had blood tests and mammograms, and I asked about repeating the bone scan but was told I did not need it. Gradually I became more comfortable with the checkups, and I am thankful that they have become less frequent.

I was living life again and loving it. However, if I ever get caught saying that life went back to "normal," I would not want that to be interpreted as meaning that it is just like it was before the cancer. I view life as being much more fragile and valuable than I did before. During my journey I lost three close friends to cancer, one of whom was my doctor, and another very close friend to a burst aorta. This has all made me that much more thankful for my survival and that of those who are still with me. About that time I had a conversation with Dr. N.

"How old are you?" I asked. We compared ages and it turns out he is 3 months younger than I am. I said, "Up to now you were Dr. N. to me; I wanted you to be in authority over me and in authority over my cancer. Now, David, I hope you will be my friend." We have been so ever since, and it has been a pleasure to work for the advancement of breast cancer care, and especially men's breast cancer care in general, and David's pioneering work in particular.

There is a role that I think cancer survivors have an obligation to play. I call it a "pastoral" role. It has to do with spreading education about cancer and helping people not to feel so helpless. I have said to every group of people whom I have had the opportunity to address, and especially to men, that when you are in the shower and you are all soapy and your skin is slippery, just keep your mind a bit alert. If you feel *anything* you don't think should be there, *have it checked out.* Do not ignore it because you are a man and you don't think you can get breast cancer. I have been on TV and radio, taken part in cancer walks, and raised money for research. But the most important thing to do is to urge people to fight back and not feel so intimidated.

I feel in this regard that I have a new power. When I talk with someone who has just been diagnosed or is going through treatment, I don't have that old awkward feeling, like cancer is this big black mystery that we can't really talk about. I used to say, "Wow, we're pulling for you," or something equally inane. That was, of course, always a sincere statement, but now when I talk with a cancer patient we are friends instantly, members of a club that is full of warmth and mutual support. We would not have chosen to join this club, but it nevertheless gives us a bond with each other that I would never have understood had I not experienced it. I immediately say, "How is your treatment going?" and "What are you taking?" and "Have you thought about doing this or that to make it easier?" And we do a lot of hugging and cheering for each other. We can't change each other's journey, which for some of us will lead back to normal life and for some of us will not, but we are on it together and we go along hand in hand, with the help of family and friends, and doctors and nurses who have new tools every day to help us.

Epilogue: What I Learned from My Patients

"Doctors have often discovered the right remedies by listening to their patients."
—"My Secret Book," by Francesco Petrarca, AD 1347.

I have learned much from reading what the breast cancer survivors wrote. I thought I knew my patients so well that there would be nothing new for me, but I was wrong. In reading stories that I didn't previously know, I discovered an innate wisdom in each of these patients. The wisdom that they expressed, individually and collectively, takes the form of six main themes:

THE EMOTIONAL VALUE OF MEDICAL INFORMATION

Medical information is important both to guide the best decisions that the patient has to make about her course of treatment and to alleviate unnecessary fears based on myths or out of date information.

Many patients in this book noticed how important it is to educate themselves about their disease. Some breast cancer patients, especially in the past, relied on their doctors to make all the important decisions for their care. They didn't look deeply into options for management because they believed that the "doctor knows best." This is analogous to building a new home without choosing the builder or reviewing the architectural plans. I remember the days when doctors were like gods and would dictate the treatment of the patient without explaining even minor details. I am glad those days are mostly gone. I no longer feel the burden of making decisions for patients. My function as a breast surgeon is to start the process of healing by educating the patient. In addition to the information I impart, patients have extensive access to all sorts of wonderful educational materials.

Information gleaned from patients has tangible benefits. Before 1990 we admitted patients to the hospital for days or weeks after breast surgery. Then we found that we could send patients home the day of their breast cancer surgery provided we were sure they understood everything that would happen before, during, and after the actual operation. Patients may choose to remain hospitalized overnight, but most prefer to go home right after surgery. Physicians and nurses provide that information before the surgery, and most patients welcome and benefit from recovery in their own homes.

Radiological screening is an important first step in gathering medical information. The long-term survival rate for breast cancer has improved progressively over the past 30 years, largely because of radiological imaging, including mammography, ultrasound, and magnetic resonance imaging (MRI). Women have become more accepting of mammograms even though they are uncomfortable and sometimes painful for a few minutes during the procedure. The compliance rates for mammography vary by geographic region and financial factors, but in some areas of the United States, the mammogram rate for women over 40 is better than 80 percent. The medical benefit of routine screening cannot be overstated, for ignorance of early cancer may lead to irreversible advanced stages of the cancer.

Many experience the anxiety of being "called back" for additional studies when initial screening tests prove inconclusive. Physicians try to accommodate the agonizing uncertainty by improving the turn around time between the initial screening mammogram and additional mammograms to focus more intensely on a new and possibly abnormal finding. In the best of all possible worlds, all of the additional studies and follow-up examinations would be done on the same day. But delays are inevitable. Sometimes emotionally vulnerable patients express anger and discouragement, feeling that "nobody cares." An important part of the "medical information" patients require is the knowledge that they are being cared for by compassionate physicians, nurses, and allied personnel. When the patient senses that healing bond it creates a feeling of trust and confidence.

Patients who undergo a needle biopsy of a breast abnormality often wait days to weeks to be seen by a surgeon. This is because a pathologist must process the tissue, a lengthy process requiring an established laboratory protocol, which cannot (and should not) be hurried. Understandably, this delay adds to the frustration of waiting for the diagnosis. Some patients are so affected by this period of uncertainty that they have difficulty sleeping. Irritability, anxiety, depression, and aggression are often exhibited in people who are normally tranquil and happy. Health care professionals can help by listening to the patient's expressions of anguish and by explaining why apparent delays may be required to facilitate an accurate diagnosis and the most beneficial course of treatment.

Contemplating a surgical procedure is never easy, and the prevalence of frightening misinformation makes it even more difficult. We remember horror stories of death, adverse effects, and complications from surgical procedures. A surprisingly common myth is the one that equates "letting the air in" during an operation with the tumor spreading more quickly. I first heard this story from my grandmother when I was a child. Scientific research has proved this to be inaccurate, but it is still a widely held misconception by the lay public.

Equally frightening is the prospect of a general anesthetic, and many fear the loss of control and the potential mortality. In the modern era, it is most unlikely that anyone will die under anesthetic, especially for operations involving surface structures like the breast. The risk is approximately one person in two million who undergo a general anesthetic in the United States. The risks are significantly higher for patients who have other major problems, such as heart, kidney, lung, or liver failure. But we always factor those comorbidities into the equation when we plan a surgical procedure in patients with breast cancer. Patients can be brought to understand these facts, and their understanding will help them master the anxieties that naturally accompany the diagnosis of a serious illness.

The surgical treatment of breast cancer has changed drastically in the past 30 years, but many patients do not know about the important improvements. The change was initiated by the introduction of the modern clinical research era of randomized trials that were started in the 1970s. These studies disproved long-established dogmas that emphasized aggressive local therapy as the key for controlling breast cancer and preventing recurrence. As a consequence, most women with early breast cancer are now able to preserve their breasts, and often undergo removal of just one sentinel lymph node in the armpit. However, many women react to the diagnosis and the planning of surgery by requesting a mastectomy. The idea is to "get rid of the organ because it is diseased; it has done its job and I don't need it any more." While a lumpectomy or partial mastectomy leaves the breast intact, some women don't want to deal with the repeated fear of recurrent cancer in that same breast, a risk of about 0.3 percent per year of remaining life, or a 30 percent chance of getting another breast cancer in 100 years. The average age of breast cancer diagnosis in the United States is about 60, so most people that age can look forward to living another 20 to 30 years. In these patients, the likelihood of getting another breast cancer in the breast is less than 10 percent. The medical profession looks at these numbers and advises breast-conserving surgery. Some patients, driven by overwhelming fear, are reluctant to follow these guidelines. Finding ways to calm one's fears can help to avoid making irreversible decisions. I wrestle with the desire to support patient autonomy, even when decisions differ from my recommendations, and the equally strong commitment to provide the safest care with the best cosmetic and functional result. Imparting useful information and helping patients grapple with strong emotions is part of my mission, but matching these activities to individual patient needs is as much an art as a science.

It isn't always easy to think rationally about data that would help make decisions, and that includes decisions about chemotherapy. Physicians use nomograms and algorithms to provide statistical justification for our recommendations. Medicine, however, is by no means a purely science-based profession, and in some instances management plans are based on the art or the experience of the health care provider. For similar reasons, patients often make decisions based on a gut feeling. These gut feelings, like the most artful management plans, need to be evaluated in the context of the best available medical knowledge.

Plans and protocols change over time. Guidelines for adjuvant systemic therapy (drugs that circulate in the blood stream and kill tumor cells in organs distant from the breast) continue to evolve. Hormonal manipulation is commonly prescribed for hormone-sensitive tumors. Tamoxifen, a synthetic drug that is very helpful in the management of selected breast cancers, has been the standard therapy for most women with hormone responsive breast cancer. However, research continues to find better ways to cure patients with breast cancer. Exciting changes have surfaced since many of the patients in our book were treated. A newer class of drugs that act in a way similar to Tamoxifen, the Aromatase inhibitors, have been shown to be better than Tamoxifen for treatment of breast cancer in postmenopausal women, although they are not useful for premenopausal women. I have learned the value of informing my patients of these developments as a way to nurture hope while providing the best treatment.

The pace of change in molecular medicine is astounding. The human genome project has opened an entirely new vista of so-called targeted therapy. There is little doubt that this will lead to better treatment for breast cancer in the future. It has also focused attention on another aspect of disease management: the enormously varied genetic makeup of patients. Drug treatment is strongly dependent on many different genes. A drug that works miraculously in one patient may work only modestly in another. For example, a commonly used anti-inflammatory and analgesic preparation, Ibuprofen, is more effective as a painkiller in women than it is in men. Patients can understand the occasional need to try different drugs in order to find the ones that work best with their own genetic makeup.

Radiation of the breast has also changed over the years. Women remember what it was like decades ago. Today's patients may have been young girls when they saw tragic and harmful effects of radiation in close relatives. One of the horror stories was the vivid remembrance of a paternal aunt who had breast cancer in the 1960s. In those days, it wasn't uncommon for breast cancer patients to have a total mastectomy and then get radiation. In this case, the aunt had two of the dreaded complications of radiation, burns of the skin and pneumonitis (scarring of the lung with a chronic cough). It is easy to understand the fear of radiation in a patient who remembers the suffering of her aunt. However, science has changed the way the radiation is delivered, and we almost never see those problems anymore.

Sometimes, we health care professionals can help patients by explaining their disease in a broader medical context. Cancer may be a chronic disease. Although patients and physicians alike would like to cure cancer, it is often better to aim for a comfortable, functional life free of distressing symptoms. Fear of the "Big C" makes most people forget that there are millions of people living with chronic diseases, like diabetes, asthma, congestive cardiac failure, or hypertension. In some cases patients with these diseases may be worse off than the average person with breast cancer. Again, as the stories in this book show, knowledge and perspective can be a great comfort to patients. Ignorance breeds fear, and fear impedes recovery.

HELPING WITH ONE'S OWN TREATMENT

Many patients newly diagnosed with breast cancer strongly consider a change in their lifestyle. It is an intuitive thought based on common logic. After all, if they got breast cancer they must have done something wrong. If their lifestyle is what caused the breast cancer then it is necessary to change. The media have helped fuel the belief that diet is a central factor in the initiation and promotion of breast cancer, and many patients change their diets, some drastically. I remember one patient who read an article on carrots and their importance in treating breast cancer. When I saw her she was orange from carotenemia, a condition caused by eating too many carrots. I was astounded at how many carrots she consumed per day. She was so passionate in her belief that she persuaded her friends to follow her example. I imagined a whole neighborhood of orange women! There is, unfortunately, no scientific proof that drastic diets of any sort are helpful in treating breast cancer. Common sense dictates that a well-balanced diet is important, which may be helpful because it encourages discipline and pours over to other lifestyle changes: getting an adequate amount of sleep, meditation, exercise, spending time with family and friends, focusing on caring relationships, taking better care of other diseases (such as hypertension and diabetes), taking supplemental vitamins and minerals if indicated, stimulating the mind and avoiding toxins. It is not necessary to make a radical change in one's diet to avoid toxins. Simple attention to eating a balanced diet, such as the types described by Dr. Andrew Weill's books, makes the most sense.

Dietary supplements are not held to the same standards as new drugs. They can be sold without a prescription in the United States. The general public regards such additional treatment as quite useful to the management of their disease. Physicians, however, are rather skeptical of their value. While detailed information is available for scientifically proven drugs, evidence-based guidance for the use of herbs and botanical agents is often lacking. The National Center for Complementary and Alternative Medicine (NCCAM) awards grants through the National Institutes of Health to do scientifically valid studies to test the claims of the added value of supplements. This will allow patients and physicians to more adequately evaluate the effectiveness of these agents. To me it is rather sobering to recognize the vast numbers of botanicals, minerals, and vitamins that are sold to patients as valuable therapeutic agents. This industry generated thirty-two billion dollars in revenue in 2004 alone. My major concern is the danger in assuming that herbs are inherently safe because they are "natural." Some products contain potentially harmful contaminants, including synthetic estrogens, which could actually promote breast cancer growth. Without scientific oversight for herbal therapies the public risks ingestion of substances that are potentially ineffective, toxic, or both.

Patients can do much to help their own treatment through constructive emotional work. The culture of North America emphasizes focusing on the positive, which is a very important part of treatment. People who are depressed, pessimistic, anxious, and fearful experience more pain than those who look at the "good side." A good attitude is an important component of healing. How does one attain such a positive attitude? It may not be easy and is certainly not like turning on a faucet. Some patients are genetically predisposed to being positive, and for them it is relatively easy to snap out of the frightening thoughts that invade the mind during all stages of breast cancer treatment. Others have to work hard to achieve an optimistic state of mind, and some may need psychological and pharmacological aids to awaken genuine hope appropriate for their particular set of circumstances.

Emotion may cloud judgment. During the restless and frenetic days that follow the diagnosis of breast cancer it is difficult to make decisions without emotion. A common reaction is for a woman to demand a mastectomy, even when a less radical operation is perfectly adequate. I find it useful to take a deep breath and discuss the options carefully. As a surgeon I worry about performing an irreversible operation that the person may later regret, even if they've undergone a reconstruction by a plastic surgeon. It is just as important to make the right decision about chemotherapy. The intensity of the emotional reaction to the diagnosis and discussion with a physician will often dissipate in a few days and allow better decisions that will better match the patient's long-term needs. Talking with nurses, social workers, and breast cancer survivors can also be very helpful.

Many stories in this book and others from my experiences in the clinic demonstrate that most patients recognize the importance of cooperation. Intuitive wisdom tells us that the health team functions better when they feel the trust of the patient. Some patients, however, revealed negative feelings about one health care professional or another. Such stories surprised me because my own perception of the same professionals, my colleagues, was often completely different.

Patients and their health care team face an interesting dilemma: we expect patients to absorb a large volume of emotionally laden new information in a short amount of time. We ask that decisions be made fairly quickly, but we also want patients to deliberate carefully using logic and perspective rather than fear as their guide. I want to accept patients' right to, and yes, their need to complain, but I honestly struggle to achieve this ideal. I am so keenly aware of the altruism in most physicians, nurses, and allied health care providers that I believe these individuals do their very best simply because they want to do so. Every now and then a patient believes that challenging the professional caregiver at every step is somehow supposed to make that person provide better treatment. I believe it does just the opposite, undermining the spirit of cooperation. Health care professionals are under constant surveillance and frequent evaluation, and we take care to "do the right thing."

Taking control of one's own breast cancer treatment really means creating a partnership with the health care professionals involved in one's treatment. No person can do her own operation, or give herself intravenous anticancer medications, or plan and execute her own radiation. But it is essential to become actively involved with the professionals giving the treatments. One can be alert to one's treatment every step of the way, ask questions, and build an effective doctor-patient relationship through open dialogue and trust.

It is important to feel comfortable with the doctor. I have frequently seen patients for a second opinion, perhaps for confirmation or to hear a broader range of options. Often the patient hopes that another physician will give them a different diagnosis. Perhaps there was a mistake. By the time a visit to a second physician is accomplished the patient has had a little time to reflect and she often comes in with a slightly different perspective. She may like the second physician better. This creates a conflict since she may feel that she should go back to the first physician. I believe that the patient should be selfish and seek medical help from personnel with whom they feel comfortable. Nothing is quite as disconcerting as to yield one's dignity and trust to someone in whom you don't have full confidence.

The many complicated medical concepts and terms that patients hear when they start their treatment can be confusing. Well-meaning friends and relatives may contribute to this confusion by coming up with all sorts of stories that they read and hear from many sources. Frankly, many of these are based on fairy tales and pseudoscience, and they should be treated as such. We physicians need to get better at communicating our concerns about the dangers of these convincing, appealing, but untrue remedies for cancer. Certainly, there is room for us to invite our patients to share their experiences and beliefs and also the sources. Open-minded dialogue is an ideal worth working toward for both doctor and patient.

Finally, one can enhance treatment by avoiding constant thoughts about cancer. I've found that patients who immerse themselves in the matters of everyday living cope better with their cancer experience. I am not recommending ignoring the seriousness of breast cancer. That would be dangerous. It is also harmful to spend every day, and all day (and night), dwelling on the illness. The human brain tends to revert to continuous thoughts and fears that have not been processed and resolved adequately. Who hasn't had the experience of trying to sleep when something difficult and worrisome cropped up during the day? Try as you might, the topic is right there in your conscious mind and you can't easily get rid of it. Fortunately, with conscious effort, humans can learn to soothe the seething mind through activity, distraction, meditation, and the like. Even when we are superb caretakers of others, we may need a little help easing our own distress. From my experience this effort is always worthwhile.

INTERPERSONAL DIFFICULTIES

After the diagnosis of breast cancer women continue to interact with spouses, children, friends, relatives, and many others, including health care professionals. It's not always easy.

I've often wondered how spouses deal with their wives experiencing breast cancer. Academic studies by psychologists and sociologists are available, but I have never had a patient discuss this difficult area directly with me. Nor did I find this topic discussed in any detail by the stories in this book. I can thus only speculate from the few direct answers to questions I've posed to husbands over my years of clinical practice. Most of the time husbands whose wives have undergone a mastectomy say it doesn't matter to them because they "love the person who is more than a breast." I can remember only two or three cases out of thousands of women I've treated where the marriage disintegrated soon after breast cancer treatment started. I did not investigate those marriages but I believe they must have been in deep trouble before the onset of the breast cancer.

Many patients feel a sense of discomfort from others who aren't quite sure how to deal with them now that they have breast cancer. People who are uncomfortable talking to cancer patients may be projecting their own fears of the disease and its potential consequences. Societal habits often inhibit open and truthful conversation. One of my patients confronted her neighbor by telling her that she was still the same person, that she hadn't contracted an infectious disease, and that she intended to continue living exactly the way she had previously lived. It's hard to know what the neighbor was thinking, but she did relax a little over time and began to accept her friend with her new situation.

Another patient of mine wasn't as fortunate. Her neighbor stopped visiting. One day they bumped into each other at the local supermarket. The meeting was embarrassing for the neighbor and puzzling for the patient. The neighbor stared at her, mumbled something uninterpretable, and walked off. The patient, a warm and loving woman in her mid 50s, was devastated. It wasn't until she discussed this with other friends and family that she realized that her neighbor could not muster the needed strength of character to deal with her friend's crisis.

THE VALUE OF SUPPORT

One of the most important things I have learned from these stories from breast cancer patients is the need to find comfort and support. For many women, a critical difficulty is in providing comfort for oneself. Women naturally tend toward nurturing others, a behavior that is essential for the survival of their children and for the species. As with other personality traits, the degree of nurturing ability varies greatly. Those who are the most nurturing, empathetic, sympathetic, and compassionate tend to be the least selfish. Compassion may be difficult when experiencing extreme tiredness after an operation under general anesthetic. It takes weeks to get over the feeling of weariness. Ideally, the only mandate for patients during this period would be to focus on one's own needs and rest. Before the modern medical era the only effective treatment physicians could prescribe was rest, an ancient remedy, many thousands of years old. We are all so used to rushing around during our daily routines that we're restless if we have to sit still for any length of time. The solution is simple, but finding ways to actually slow down and nurture oneself can be challenging. If you really pay attention to your body, you will know when it is time to start an active life again.

Friends and family can provide necessary support. They can drive patients to appointments, cook meals, be a shoulder to cry on, provide emotional comfort, administer medications, change dressings, and help with other daily requirements. The stress most people feel during their breast cancer treatments can hinder their ability to process information. Many rely on spouses, family, and friends to reinforce what they heard in the doctor's office. It is amazing what patients hear when they first get the diagnosis of breast cancer. Two sets of ears are better than one, and three sets may be even better. When they get home the patient and spouse can discuss what they heard and come up with rational decisions regarding management.

Comfort and support frequently come from health care workers. Everyone with breast cancer would like a surgeon similar to the one that treated Pam as described in Chapter 1. How marvelous it would be to have your surgeon come to your house to give you the diagnosis and discuss your treatment options in your own living room. Most will, however, experience the same level of dedication as expressed through an encouraging voice, a compassionate touch, a willingness to listen, a timely joke, or any of the many other ways that people find to support one another. Research from Harold Koenig, M.D., a psychiatrist at Duke University in Durham, North Carolina, has shown that patients who feel cared for are likely to recover better from their disease. I encourage patients to tune into and appreciate expressions of support, whatever the source.

Support can take the form of a powerful personal connection. One patient, a Scot from Glasgow, wrote a brief essay that reminded me vividly of the day we first met. She was scared because her husband had been diagnosed with breast cancer and was not doing well. Somewhere deep inside her she wanted to know "the truth" about her own newly diagnosed breast cancer. She raised herself up to her full five feet and two inches, and looked at me through her thick glasses. I had just described in great detail the planned treatment. I felt as if she were searching the very depths of my subconscious mind for the truth. She had a delightful accent, one quite unique to her city of origin.

"Now, you're not going to hurt me, are you, doctor?"

"Of course not," I assured her.

"Well, if you do, I'll be forced to give you a Glasgow kiss."

"What's a Glasgow kiss?"

Her expression was both gleeful and impish. She grabbed hold of the lapels of my white coat, pulled my neck and head downward with a sudden and surprising strength, and pushed her forehead into mine. I was stunned while she grinned triumphantly. Apparently, this was a common method of punishment by street gangs in the Glasgow of her childhood. With this simple story and single gesture my patient communicated her sense of humor, individual strength, connection to her cultural community, her fears, her bond with me as physician, and so much more. These moments of connection are among the most satisfying of my clinical day.

Many people have cancer and one would never know. One of my patients, determined to keep working through her treatments, broke down one day and cried in her office. Her coworkers gathered around her and listened to her saga. She soon heard three of them confide that they, too, had experienced the same diagnosis and treatment, and they rallied to help a new "sister." She was amazed. They looked so "normal." They managed their lives without making a big deal of their disease, a tribute to their strength, dignity, resolve, and determination. Silence, however, exacts a price because it makes patients invisible and places them beyond the reach of help from others.

VARIETIES OF FAITH

We've said earlier that it is important to take charge of the scientific aspects of one's treatment. But there is a fine balance between what one can influence by doing things to help overcome the disease, and "letting go and letting God." Research shows that faith and spirituality contribute to healing, too. A patient obviously needs to have faith in the health care professionals, but here we are focused on a different faith, one that has various definitions and meanings for different individuals. Belief in the God of Abraham is a powerful support system for Christians, Jews, and Muslims. But faith takes many different forms. I've seen the pagan faith of the Bushmen of Southern Africa performing ritual dances and achieving a trance-like state prior to hunting expeditions. Such is the power of belief that Bushmen glean courage from this faith and are probably better able to tolerate the harsh circumstances they endure while hunting in the wild. Other examples of faith occur when absorbing the wonders of nature, perhaps by walking in the park, or in a river valley, or on a beautiful beach. A spiritual experience may be as simple as listening to music, drinking a good cup of coffee, or a walk in the garden, or stroking a pet.

Though details vary, most religions invest in rituals and prayers that address illness, including how to deal emotionally with the acute stress invoked by being ill. Sadly, many individuals are unfamiliar with even their own religions' views on sickness, healing, and health.

Whatever the source, faith enhances one's ability to see clearly and to find a comfortable place with one's thoughts. The bottom line, though, is we all need to be in a caring environment in times of stress. Faith, when paired with reason, is like radar that sees through the fog. There is so much that is unfamiliar, unsettling, and uncertain in cancer care. Faith helps because, as Martin Luther King said, "Faith is taking the first step even when you don't see the whole staircase."

Should one expect spiritual support from one's doctor? Harold Koenig, in his recent book *Spirituality in Patient Care,* reports many components that guide us in answering this question. Less than one in ten doctors asks a patient about their faith and religious beliefs. Doctors feel uncomfortable about broaching this topic with their patients. Yet 70 percent of patients would like their doctors to incorporate their religious beliefs into their treatment. Ten percent would like their doctors to pray with them. Many studies support the idea that religious people have better health outcomes than those who claim no religious affiliations or beliefs. Two-thirds of American medical schools now offer courses on spirituality to their students. With this surge in academic interest, the reluctance of doctors to use this in their practices may decrease over time.

I am amazed that some patients, in the very midst of their own problems, think about others worse off than they are. Some years ago I treated a patient with terminal cancer who was repeatedly admitted to the hospital. She had many rounds of chemotherapy and surgery and was in constant pain and discomfort. Her life had been disrupted by her disease, and the health team watched her carefully for signs of depression. She didn't complain and seemed to be happy. She would walk around the hospital corridors, greeting other patients, nurses, orderlies, janitors, food handlers, volunteers, and visitors. She always smiled graciously, even though I knew she was in severe pain. Most remarkable of all her activities was her introducing herself to patients who were admitted for treatment. She sat at the bedside of one particular young woman with a rare tumor, talking to her for hours on end. I discovered my patient was giving this young woman a message of hope and faith. I'm convinced she accomplished a lot for other patients, and I'm equally certain that this activity helped her deal with her own disease.

Not everyone can give of themselves emotionally or physically to help another patient directly. But it is possible to help other patients that are not known to you at the time of your treatment. Some of my patients tell about volunteering for research protocols. Some expressed their hope that this might help other patients, perhaps even their own children and grandchildren. Pam Brady, despite her own illness, felt the need to comfort others whose illnesses may have been worse than her own. Belief in the sanctity of life, the value of one's fellow humans, the need to help others, gratefulness, forgiveness, and the love that these thoughts and activities engender comprise the core of religious faith and humanitarianism.

We naturally aspire to joy. Ludwig von Beethoven, whose biographers describe him as a violent, angry, antisocial man, prone to rages and vituperous language, and suffering from lead poisoning, wrote the most wonderful music. Despite the agony of being deaf, he wrote his 9th Symphony, a triumph of the spirit and a tribute to the tendency of humans to look for the light and good in each other. There are many examples in art, literature, music, sport, science, and human interactions of wonderful accomplishments at times of great suffering and pain. We don't have to be totally at peace with ourselves to connect with our giving, loving, and spiritual side.

FEAR AND COURAGE

Loss of control is a deeply human fear, especially for patients newly diagnosed with breast cancer. Because they associate the "Big C" with death, most patients believe that they will die from the disease. However, the truth is most people with early stage breast cancer don't die of this disease. Nevertheless, the sense of impending loss is common. People recently diagnosed with breast cancer feel the progressive encroachment on their freedom by a succession of professionals who decide when and what their next course of treatment will be. It is like going into a dark tunnel and the feeling lasts for 6 to 8 months. The fear is also related to the unknown. Will they lose their dignity? Will they be able to enjoy their usual pleasures of everyday life? What about pain and other undesirable symptoms? The uncertainty directly related to the disease itself is bad enough. In addition, there is a fear of losing loved ones, and particularly a concern about ones children, pets, spouse, and friends. Working women fear loss of a job. The stories in this book show some of the many ways of working through this fear.

Courage and tenacity are personality traits expressed in many of the stories, and they certainly help when a patient experiences diagnostic procedures, surgery, chemotherapy, radiation therapy, and hormonal manipulation for months on end. It takes courage to complete the course of treatment, and I am grateful to read the many stories of brave women who have doggedly continued their lives despite the difficulties in their treatment schedules. I've learned from these women, some of whom are mothers who have managed to continue caring for their children and families despite their own difficulties. I've noticed that many women continue to work at their usual jobs despite feeling a little "under the weather." This is an exhibition of strength; a powerful reserve that seems to exist in all of us and that emerges at times of stress.

Male breast cancer patients exhibit another type of courage. Unlike women, who are constantly reminded that breast cancer is a possibility, most men don't know that the disease can strike men occasionally. Usually, the loss of a breast for a male doesn't have the same emotional weight as it does for a woman, for a man does not regard his breasts as part of his sexuality. However, there are special issues for men, who don't deal with diseases as women do. The very idea of having a "woman's disease" is anathema to a masculine mindset. It requires courage for a man to stand up in public and declare that he is a breast cancer survivor. But the most important emotional aspect of this cancer in men is that it is no less a threat to life than in women, and therefore the fears and experiences of the management practices apply equally well to them.

For many patients, and for me, every day is a blessing. We should all realize this without the "wake up call" of breast cancer. A daily ritual in some cultures is to awaken and give thanks for having awakened to another fine day. Part of that ritual in Orthodox Judaism, for example, includes thanking God for allowing you to awaken with your vision, hearing, other bodily functions intact, and your ability to be able to express your thanks. Pamela Brady is obviously grateful that she is alive. Hers is an optimistic spirit, a soul that is relatively untroubled even with her disease. William James divided human beings into two kinds: those with cheerful souls and those with sick souls. Those that are cheerful have a tendency to see things optimistically, a trait that Pam enjoys. Sick souls cannot contemplate nature and enjoy the spectacle. It is possible to work hard at one's pessimism and depression in the face of illness, but this may require professional help, either psychological or spiritual, or a combination of the two. As many of the stories in this book suggest, most patients can find many ways to get the support needed.

It has been a great privilege to learn from my patients. Reading their stories has enriched my clinical practice, and I am certain that I approach each new patient with a greater wisdom. Even though I haven't directly experienced the stresses, emotions, and feelings of a patient going through the cycles of breast cancer treatment, I can certainly experience the ordinary miracles of courage and hope that are evident in each of their stories.

INDEX

About the Author

S. DAVID NATHANSON, M.D., is a Breast Surgical Oncologist and Director of Breast Care Services in the Department of Surgery at Henry Ford Health System in Detroit, Michigan. He is the author of some 200 journal articles and book chapters.